Disinfection of Viruses

Edited by Raymond W. Nims
and M. Khalid Ijaz

Published in London, United Kingdom

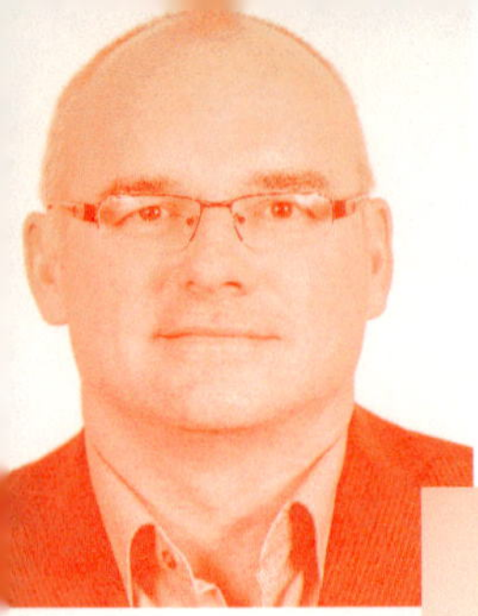
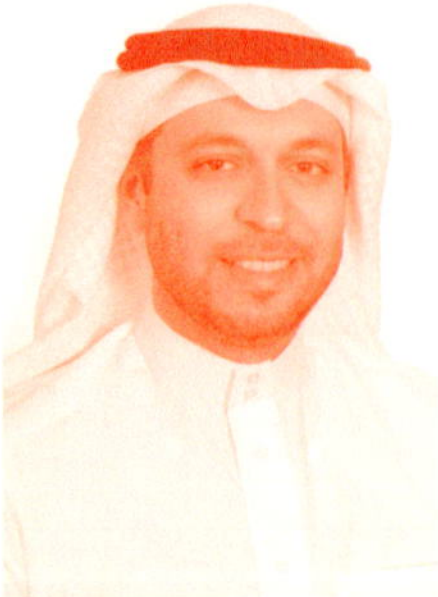
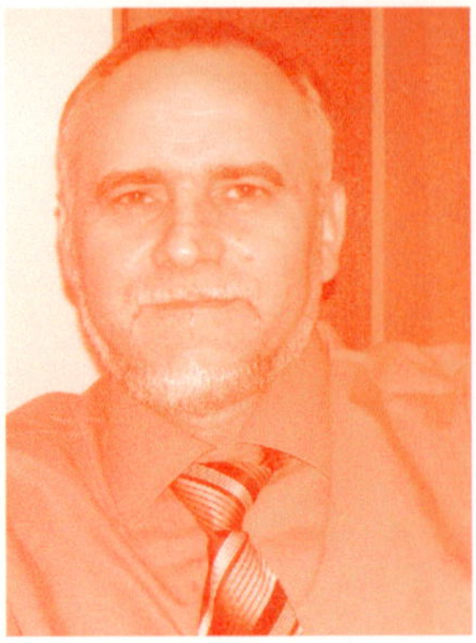
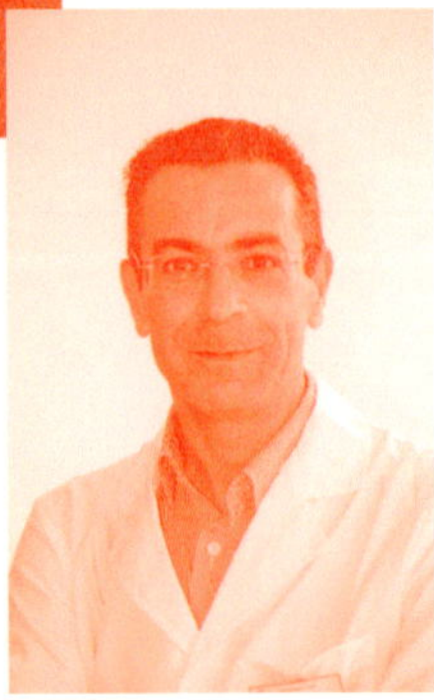
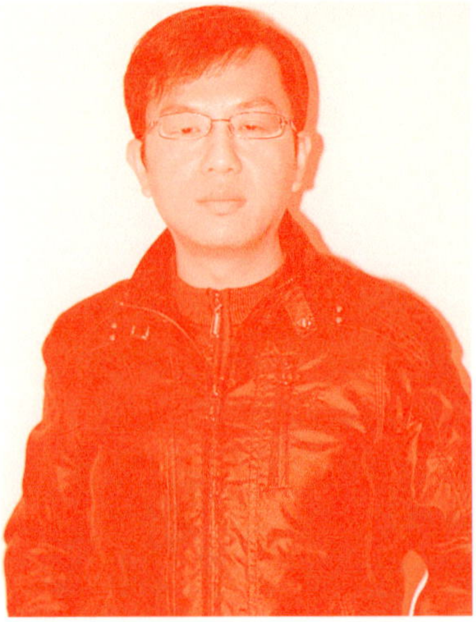
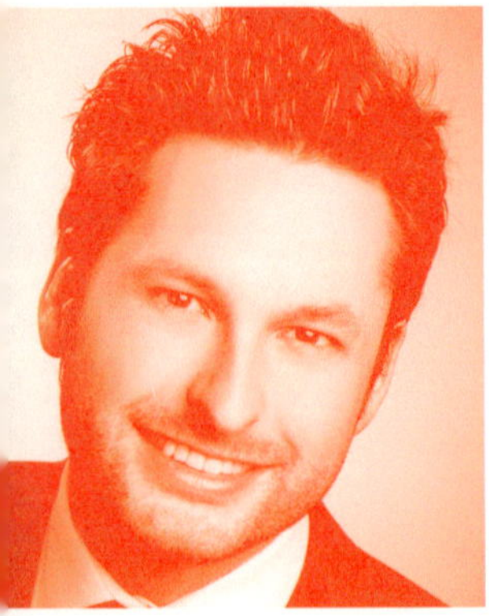
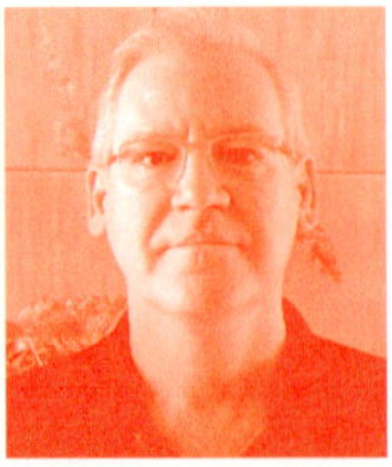

IntechOpen

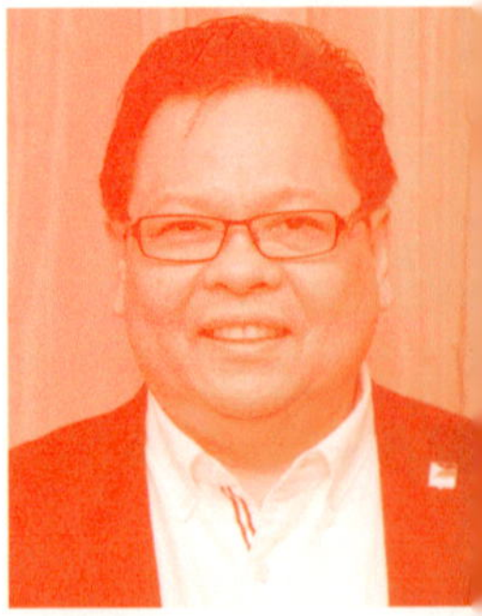
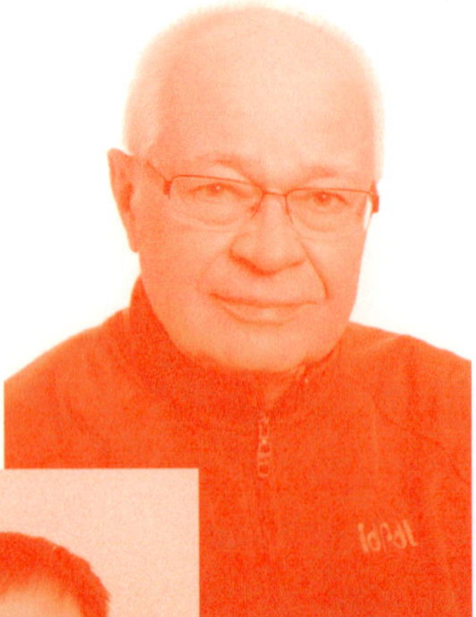
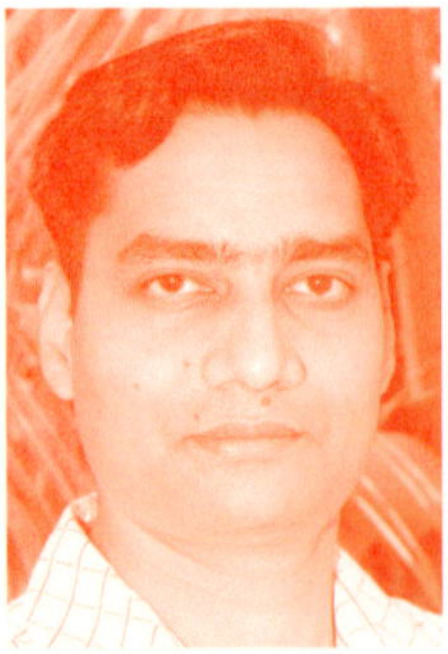
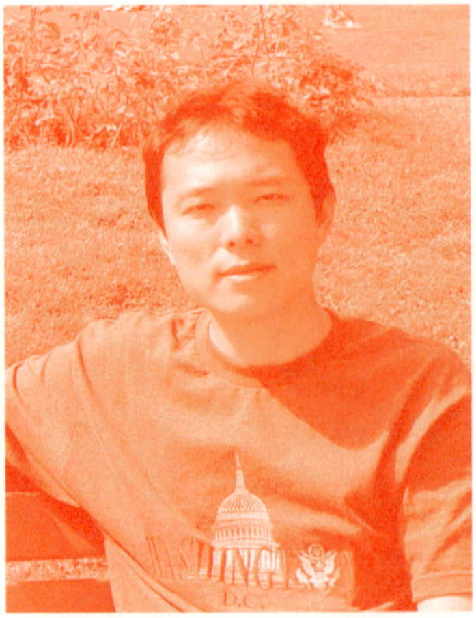
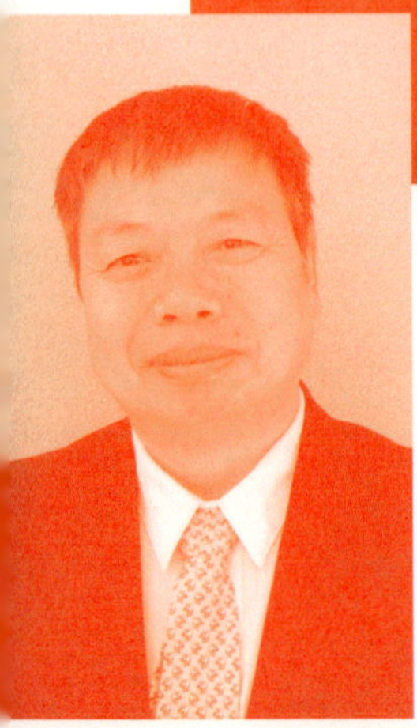
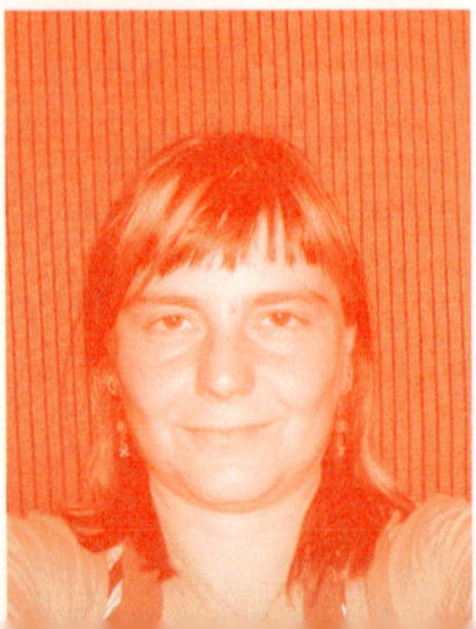

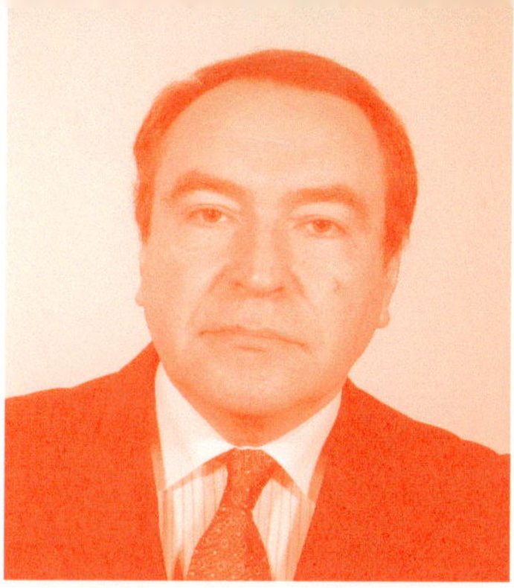
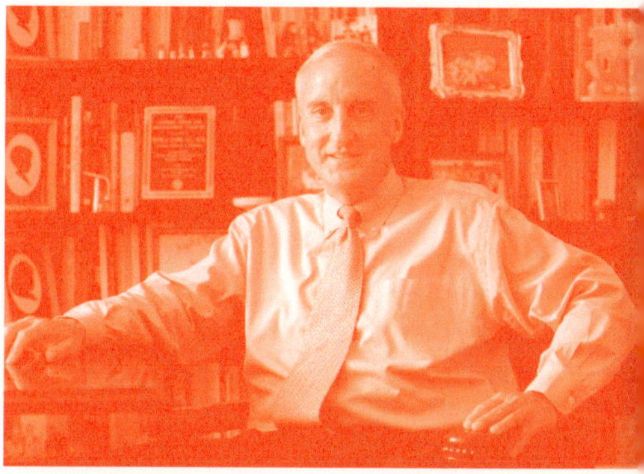
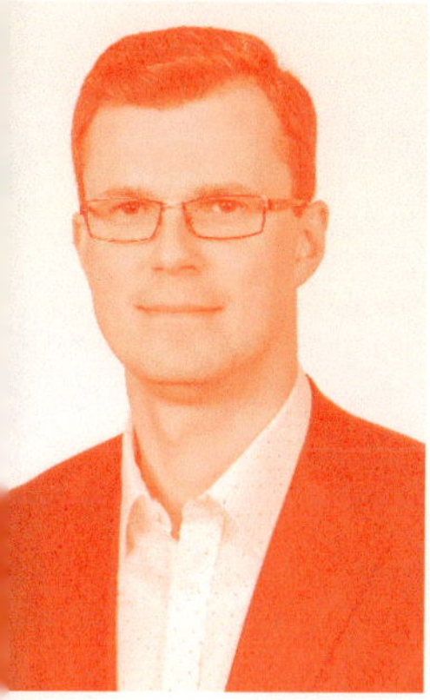
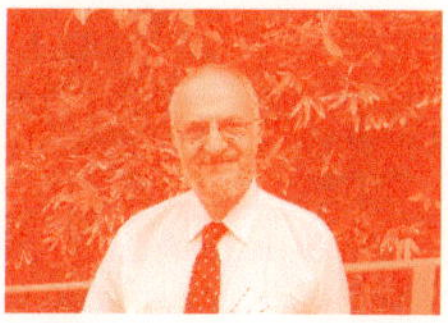
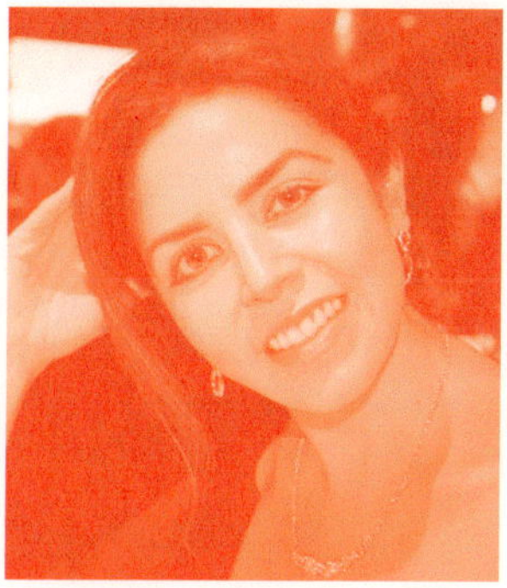

Supporting open minds since 2005

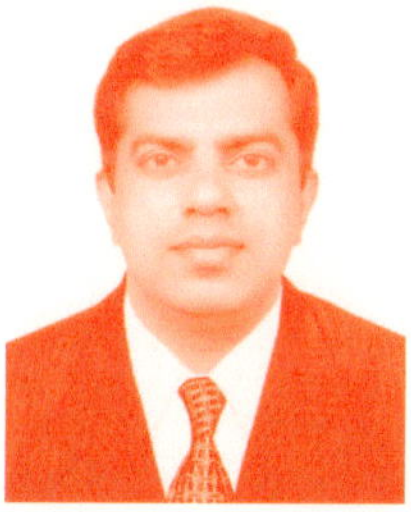
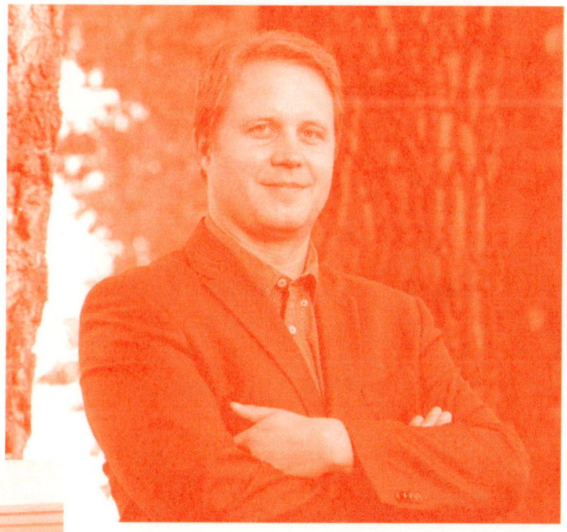
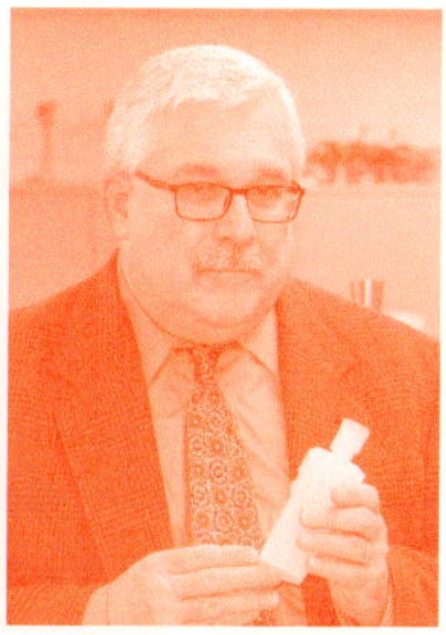
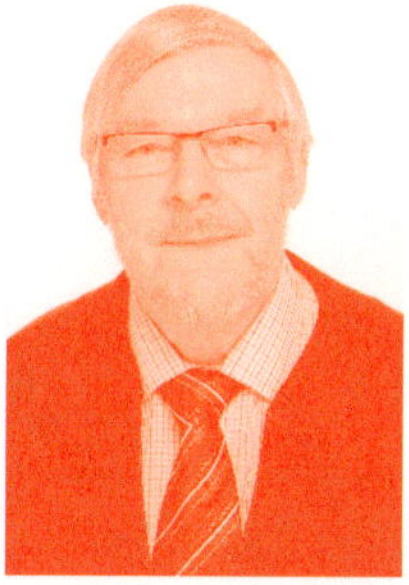
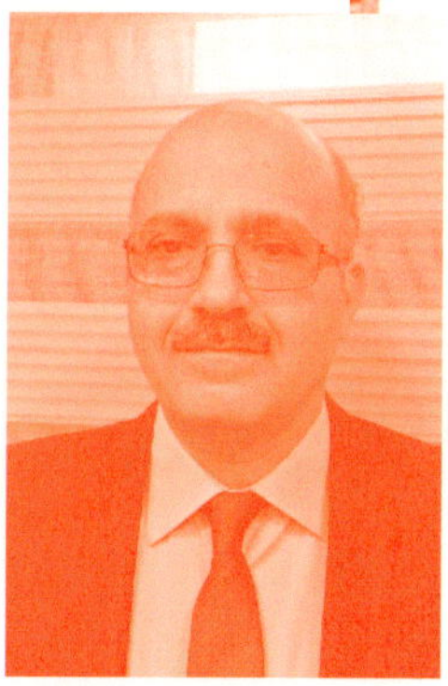
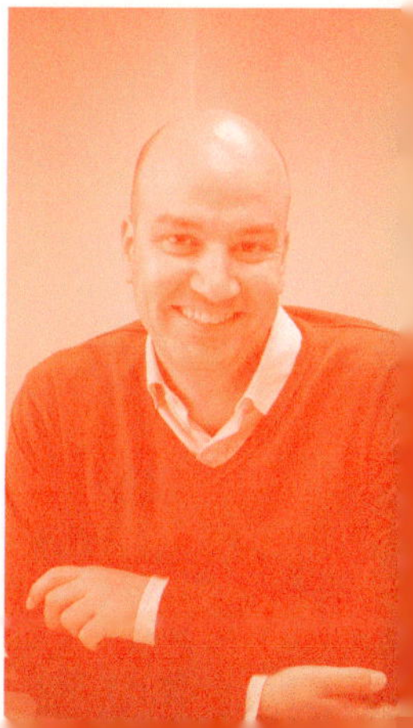
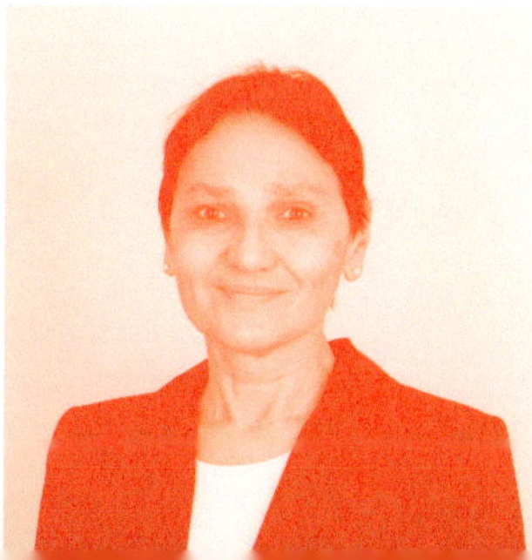

Disinfection of Viruses
http://dx.doi.org/10.5772/intechopen.95703
Edited by Raymond W. Nims and M. Khalid Ijaz

Contributors
Raymond W. Nims, Mark Plavsic, Meaghan Hislop, John R. Henneman, Frances Grinstead, Koushlesh Ranjan, Chris Lee, Charles P. Gerba, Luisa A. Ikner, Sifang Steve Zhou, Yutaka Nishihara, Hideo Eguchi, M. Khalid Ijaz, Todd A. Cutts, Julie McKinney

First published in London, United Kingdom, 2022 by IntechOpen
IntechOpen is the global imprint of INTECHOPEN LIMITED, registered in England and Wales, registration number: 11086078, 5 Princes Gate Court, London, SW7 2QJ, United Kingdom
Printed in Croatia

British Library Cataloguing-in-Publication Data
A catalogue record for this book is available from the British Library

Additional hard and PDF copies can be obtained from orders@intechopen.com

Disinfection of Viruses
Edited by Raymond W. Nims and M. Khalid Ijaz
p. cm.
Print ISBN 978-1-83962-415-5
Online ISBN 978-1-83962-416-2
eBook (PDF) ISBN 978-1-83962-417-9

For EU product safety concerns:
IN TECH d.o.o., Prolaz Marije Krucifikse Kozulić 3, 51000 Rijeka, Croatia, info@intechopen.com or visit our website at intechopen.com.

Meet the editors

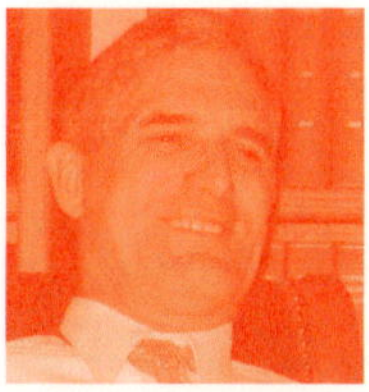

Raymond Nims has more than 37 years of experience in the biomedical sciences. He currently provides consulting services as an employee of RMC Pharmaceutical Solutions. From 2006 to 2009, Dr. Nims served in Amgen's corporate quality control group, providing subject matter expertise in viral and mycoplasma testing of raw materials and products, and serving as business process owner for Amgen's global contract analytical testing lab outsourcing program. From 1994 to 2006, he directed laboratories at BioReliance, performing viral safety, endotoxin, and cell-line identity studies for biologics cell-line characterization, raw material testing, and product lot release testing. From 1985 to 1994, he served as a chemist at the National Cancer Institute's Laboratory of Chemical Carcinogenesis. Dr. Nims obtained a Ph.D. in Chemistry (Chemical Toxicology) at The American University, Washington, DC, in 1993. He currently serves on the editorial board for *BioProcessing Journal* and has served on the ad hoc advisory boards for USP chapters 1237, 1050, and 1050.1. He is a generalist in the biomedical sciences, with a publication list spanning a wide range of topics in chemistry, carcinogenesis, biochemistry, pharmacology, toxicology, and virology.

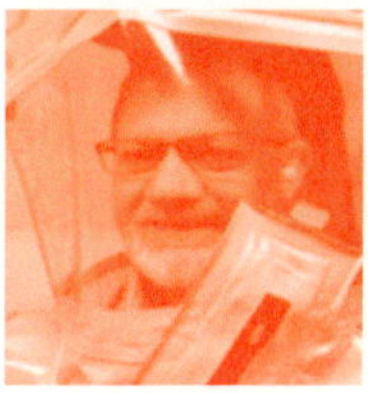

Dr. M. Khalid Ijaz is currently a Senior Research Fellow and Director of Scientific Affairs at Global Research & Development for Lysol and Dettol, Reckitt Benckiser LLC (RB). He obtained his DVM and MSc (Honors) from the Faculty of Veterinary Science, University of Agriculture, Faisalabad, Pakistan, and his Ph.D. in Microbiology and Immunology (Environmental Virology) from the University of Ottawa, Canada. He did post-doctoral work in immunobiology/vaccinology with Dr. Lorne A. Babiuk at the Vaccines and Infectious Disease Organization (VIDO), University of Saskatchewan, Canada. His research focuses over the years have included aerobiology studies on enteric and respiratory viruses (human coronavirus, rhinovirus, rotavirus, and polioviruses), and interruption of the chain of infection of human pathogens via the environment and hands through targeted use of surface and hand hygiene agents. More recently, Dr. Ijaz's research interests have included the efficacy of microbicidal actives for inactivating World Health Organization priority list viruses, including human coronaviruses (SARS-CoV, MERS-CoV, and SARS-CoV-2), the filovirus Ebola virus, the arenavirus Lassa virus, and the paramyxovirus Nipah virus.

Contents

Preface

The ongoing (as of April 4, 2022) pandemic of severe acute respiratory syndrome coronavirus 2 (SARS-CoV-2) continues to engage the infection prevention and control (IPAC) and research communities. To date, the pandemic has resulted in 492 million cases globally and more than 6 million deaths [1]. As might be expected, the pandemic has resulted in an unprecedented volume of publications on IPAC topics for this virus and its associated disease, COVID-19. As such, we thought that a collection of articles on viral disinfection might be timely. First, a little background. Viruses are not capable of reproducing themselves. Animal viruses, for instance, require a eukaryotic host cell to propagate and produce progeny. As a result, viruses are not considered "alive" or "dead"; rather, they simply are infectious or non-infectious. Disinfection of viruses is intended to render the viruses non-infectious (i.e., inactivate them), and the terms "virucidal efficacy" and "efficacy of viral inactivation" are commonly employed to denote the capability of a chemical disinfectant (e.g., alcohol) or a physical approach (e.g., ultraviolet light) for rendering a virus non-infectious. The most straightforward way to express virucidal inactivation efficacy is to state the $\log_{10}$ reduction in titer for the virus from the initial state to the post-treatment state. A commonly sought goal for an effective viral disinfectant (virucide) is to achieve at least a 3-$\log_{10}$ inactivation [2]. This equates to rendering 99.9% of the initial virus population non-infectious [3]. Of course, a 3-$\log_{10}$ virucidal efficacy, by itself, does not ensure safety under every circumstance [4], as this may depend on the initial virus titer, the human infectious dose (reported to be as low as 10 $TCID_{50}$/mL for SARS-CoV-2 [5]), susceptibility factors for the host, and the lethality of the contaminating virus. However, it is very important to note that when one describes virucidal effectiveness for a chemical disinfectant or a physical approach, one must be specific about the exact virus being disinfected (as efficacy may vary for different viruses), and the approach for disinfection (i.e., disinfection in liquid suspension, disinfection of surfaces, sanitization of hands, etc.). In addition, for many disinfection approaches, other factors come into play. These may include temperature, pH, relative humidity, presence of associated organic (soil) load, and contact time. Descriptions of virucidal efficacy, therefore, must include all this information for maximal utility to readers.

Disinfection is an important part of infection prevention and control. Most importantly, sanitization of hands and disinfection of liquids and surfaces is intended to interrupt the chain of infection, through the intermediacy of the hand, from an infected individual to an otherwise healthy individual, as depicted in **Figure 1**.

The term "targeted disinfection" is employed when chemical disinfectants or physical agents are applied strategically to high-risk surfaces (high-touch environmental surfaces [HITES]) (**Figure 2**), thereby avoiding indiscriminate use of disinfectants/agents and adverse impacts on the microbiome of the built environment [4].

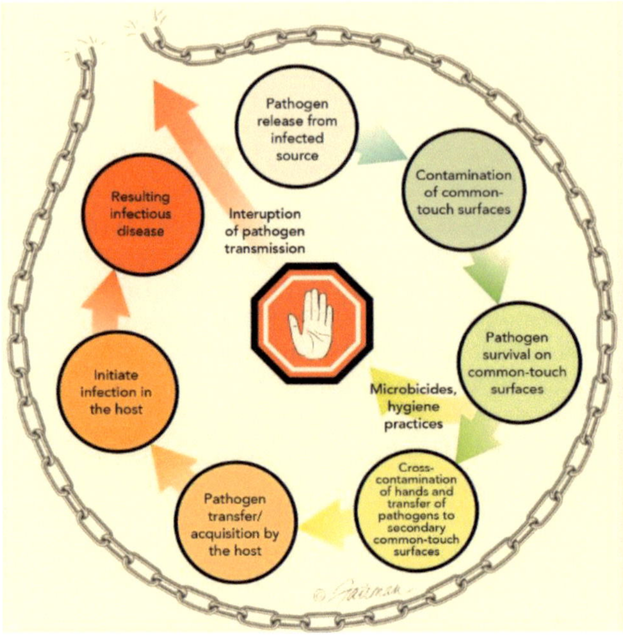
Pathogen release from infected source
Contamination of common-touch surfaces
Pathogen survival on common-touch surfaces
Cross-contamination of hands and transfer of pathogens to secondary common-touch surfaces
Pathogen transfer/ acquisition by the host
Initiate infection in the host
Resulting infectious disease
Interuption of pathogen transmission
Microbicides, hygiene practices

Figure 1.
Interrupting the chain of infection using targeted disinfection/sanitization (hygiene) approaches (from Scott et al. [4]).

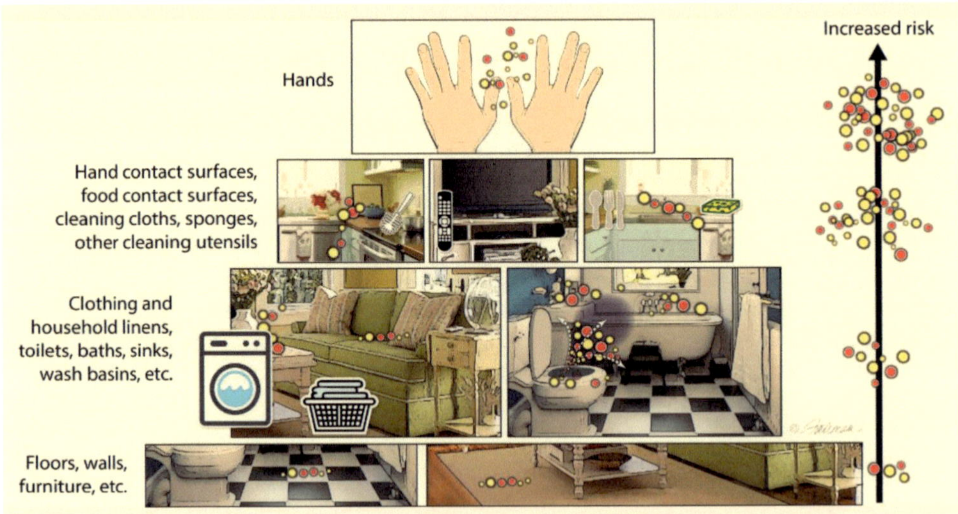

Figure 2.
High-risk surfaces and activities for viral spread to the hand, leading potentially to risk of infection dissemination to a susceptible host (from Scott et al. [4]).

Disinfection approaches are not only used for IPAC in healthcare settings and in everyday settings (homes, community, workplaces, etc.) specifically, but are also used in the pharmaceutical/biopharmaceutical industries for cleaning surfaces, disinfecting liquid waste, as barrier treatments for pathogen reduction in raw materials and process streams, and for "viral clearance" inactivation steps to assure the viral safety of products. In addition, disinfection is used in laboratory settings to render biological specimens safe for handling.

A common theme that runs throughout this book (*Disinfection of Viruses*), either implicitly or explicitly, is the concept of the hierarchy of pathogen susceptibility to microbicides. This concept was first developed by E.H. Spaulding [6], further refined by M. Klein and A. Deforest [7], S.A. Sattar [8], M.K. Ijaz and J.R. Rubino [9], and eventually incorporated into regulatory guidance by the US Environmental Protection Agency (US EPA) [10, 11]. The concept is based on the observation that different classes of pathogens differ with respect to their relative susceptibilities to the inactivating effects of chemical microbicidal active ingredients. In the most recent version of the hierarchy, infectious proteins (prions) represent the least susceptible of pathogens, while the other extreme (most susceptible) is represented by enveloped viruses (**Figure 3**). The utility of this concept, recognized by the US EPA and implemented in several guidance documents [e.g., 10, 11], is that it enables predictions to be made as to the types of microbicidal actives that might be expected to inactivate (render non-infectious) an emerging pathogen.

The US EPA's Emerging Viral Pathogens Policy was activated during the 2009 H1N1 influenza A virus pandemic [12], during the 2015 Ebola virus outbreak [13], and again in response to the SARS-CoV-2/COVID-19 pandemic in 2020 [14].

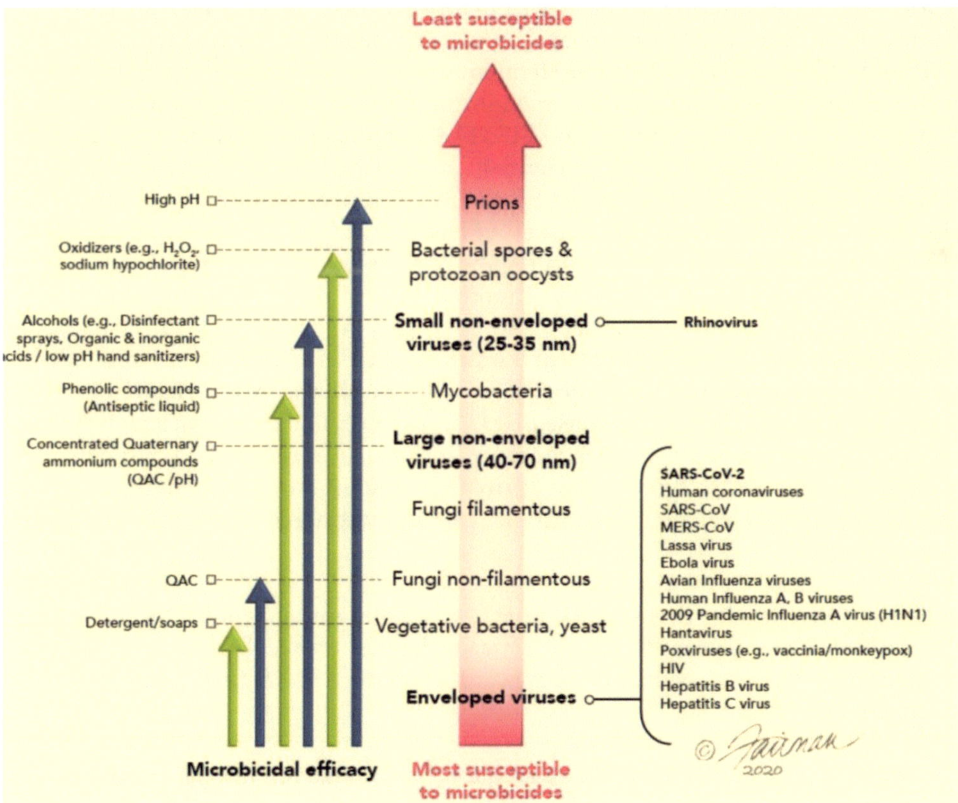

Figure 3.
Hierarchy of susceptibility of pathogens to microbicidal active ingredients ([15] modified from Sattar [8]).

Why is this important? It takes time (1) to isolate the wild-type pathogen, such as a novel virus, from the field and establish a laboratory culture; (2) to prepare stocks of the emerging pathogen to be made available to the research community; and (3) for the research community to conduct the studies needed to confirm the expected inactivation efficacy of various types of microbicides. For especially lethal pathogens, such as hemorrhagic fever viruses, only BSL-3 or BSL-4 laboratories may be capable of performing such activities. During the intervening period of time between emergence of a novel pathogen and the confirmation of inactivation efficacy of available microbicides, the US EPA guidance, based on the pathogen susceptibility hierarchy concept and virucidal efficacy data available for other variants, other family members, or appropriate surrogate pathogens, facilitates decision making on the types of microbicidal actives that will be useful in disinfecting surfaces and solutions, and sanitizing hands in the face of the novel pathogen outbreak.

Each of the chapters in this book touches on virucidal efficacy for the SARS-CoV-2 virus or enveloped viral surrogates. Per the pathogen susceptibility hierarchy concept, SARS-CoV-2, an enveloped virus of the *Coronaviridae* family, is expected to be susceptible to all classes of microbicides [15]. Evidence of this is provided within the various chapters of this book.

Section 1: "Microbicides for Viral Inactivation," contains three primary reports and three review articles. In Chapter 1, Nishihara et al. describe [16] the efficacy of a silver ion formulation for inactivating SARS-CoV-2, and the non-enveloped feline calicivirus (used as a surrogate for human norovirus), in suspension studies. In Chapter 2 [17], Lee and Henneman discuss a "Dry Hydrogen Peroxide" approach for inactivating the enveloped influenza A (H1N1) virus, and the non-enveloped feline calicivirus and MS2 bacteriophage, on surfaces or in air. In Chapter 3, Hislop, Grinstead, and Henneman describe [18], a "Hybrid Hydrogen Peroxide" approach for inactivating SARS-CoV-2, as well as a variety of other enveloped and non-enveloped viruses and bacteriophage, on surfaces. Chapter 4 [19], by Ikner and Gerba, provides a review of the efficacy of antiviral surface coatings for inactivating SARS-CoV-2 and a variety of other enveloped and non-enveloped viruses. In Chapter 5, Ijaz et al. [20] take advantage of the pathogen susceptibility hierarchy concept to predict the virucidal efficacy of microbicides against emerging and re-emerging viruses called out in the World Health Organization's 2021 Priority Disease List [21], then review the empirical data for virucidal efficacy of microbicides for the specific viruses mentioned in the list. Finally, Chapter 6 [22], by S.S. Zhou, provides a review and commentary on the application of the pathogen susceptibility hierarchy concept to the non-enveloped class of viruses.

Section 2: "Physical Inactivation Approaches," begins with Chapter 7 by Nims and Plavsic [23]. This chapter reviews the efficacy data for physical approaches (gamma irradiation, UVC irradiation, and heat) for inactivating SARS-CoV-2 and other coronaviruses.

Section 3: "Viral Persistence and Disinfection," includes a review and commentary in Chapter 8 by K. Ranjan [24] of the data on viral persistence for SARS-CoV-2 on porous and non-porous surfaces, and in liquids and air, as these data inform the need for and the approaches that might be used for disinfection of environmental surfaces, air, and wastewater in healthcare and non-healthcare settings.

The editors appreciate the time taken by the various authors to contribute to this book. It is hoped that the assembled articles will provide value to the IPAC, research, and pharmaceutical/biopharmaceutical communities during the ongoing SARS-CoV-2 pandemic and during future viral outbreaks, which undoubtedly will occur! The editors also appreciate the patient assistance of the staff at IntechOpen, Zrinka Tomicic, Kristina Kardum Cvitan, and Lucija Tomicic-Dromgool.

Raymond W. Nims, Ph.D.
RMC Pharmaceutical Solutions, Inc.,
Longmont, CO, USA

M. Khalid Ijaz, DVM, MSc (Honors), Ph.D., FRSPH
Global Research and Development for Lysol and Dettol,
Reckitt Benckiser LLC,
Montvale, NJ, USA

References

[1] Johns Hopkins University of Medicine. Coronavirus Resource Center. https://coronavirus.jhu.edu/

[2] U.S. Environmental Protection Agency. Product Performance Test Guidelines OCSPP 810.2200: Disinfectants for Use on Hard Surfaces – Efficacy Data Recommendations. 2012. https://www.regulations.gov/document?D=EPA-HQ-OPPT-2009-0150-0021

[3] Bio Technics Ltd. Log Reductions – a Beginner's Guide. 2017; https://www.endurocide.com/news/log-reductions-a-beginners-guide-2/

[4] Scott E, Bruning E, Ijaz MK. Targeted decontamination of environmental surfaces in everyday settings. In: McDonnell, Hansen, editors. Block's Disinfection, Sterilization, and Preservation. 6th edition: Wolters Kluwer, Philadelphia, 2020; pp. 960-978.

[5] Killingley B, Mann A, Kalinova M, Boyers A, Goonawardane N, Zhou J, et al. Safety, tolerability and viral kinetics during SARS-CoV-2 human challenge. Research Square. 2022. https://doi.org/10.21203/rs.3.rs-1121993/v1

[6] Spaulding EH. Chemical disinfection of medical and surgical materials. In: Block SS, editor. Disinfection, Sterilization, & Preservation, 3rd Edition: Lea & Febiger, Philadelphia, 1968.

[7] Klein M, Deforest A. Principles of viral inactivation. In: Block SS, editor. Disinfection, sterilization, and preservation, 3rd edition: Philadelphia: Lea and Febiger; 1983; pp. 422-434.

[8] Sattar SA. Hierarchy of susceptibility of viruses to environmental surface disinfectants: a predictor of activity against new and emerging viral pathogens. Journal of the AOAC International. 2007;**90**(6);1655-1658.

[9] Ijaz MK, Rubino JR. Should test methods for disinfectants use vertebrate virus dried on carriers to advance virucidal claims? Infection Control and Hospital Epidemiology. 2008;**29**(2):192-194.

[10] U.S. Environmental Protection Agency. Emerging Viral Pathogen Guidance for Antimicrobial Pesticides. 2021. https://www.epa.gov/pesticide-registration/emerging-viral-pathogen-guidance-antimicrobial-pesticides.

[11] U.S. Environmental Protection Agency. Guidance to Registrants: Process for Making Claims against Emerging Viral Pathogens not on EPA-registered Disinfectant Labels. 2016. https://www.epa.gov/sites/default/files/2016-09/documents/emerging_viral_pathogen_program_guidance_final_8_19_16_001_0.pdf

[12] U.S. Environmental Protection Agency. Guidance for Testing and Labeling Claims against Pandemic 2009 H1N1 Influenza A Virus (Formerly called Swine Flu). https://archive.epa.gov/pesticides/oppad001/web/html/h1n1-guide.html

[13] U.S. Environmental Protection Agency. Guidance to Companies on Referring to Registered Disinfectant Products that Meet the CDC Criteria for Use Against the Ebola Virus. https://archive.epa.gov/pesticides/oppad001/web/html/ebola-efficacy-claims.html

[14] U.S. Environmental Protection Agency . EPA Expands COVID-19 Disinfectant List. https://www.epa.gov/newsreleases/epa-expands-covid-19-disinfectant-list

[15] Ijaz MK, Nims RW, Zhou SS, Whitehead K, Srinivasan V,

Kapes T, et al. Microbicidal actives with virucidal efficacy against SARS-CoV-2 and other beta- and alpha-coronaviruses and implications for future emerging coronaviruses and other enveloped viruses. Scientific Reports. 2021;**11**.5626. https://doi.org/10.1038/s41598-021-84842-1

[16] Nishihara Y, Eguchi H, Zhou S. Silver ion (Ag+) formulations with virudical efficacy against severe acute respiratory syndrome coronavirus 2 (SARS-CoV-2). In: Disinfection of Viruses. Intech Open, London, UK. 2022; DOI: 10.5772/intechopen.100268

[17] Lee C, Henneman JR. Dry hydrogen peroxide for viral inactivation. In: Disinfection of Viruses. Intech Open, London, UK. 2022; DOI: 10.5772/intechopen.100451

[18] Hislop M, Grinstead F, Henneman JR. Hybrid hydrogen peroxide for viral disinfection. In: Disinfection of Viruses. Intech Open, London, UK. 2022; DOI: 10.5772/intechopen.100237

[19] Ikner LA, Gerba CP. Antiviral coatings as continuously active disinfectants. In: Disinfection of Viruses. Intech Open, London, UK. 2022; DOI: 10.5772/intechopen.101752

[20] Ijaz MK, Nims RW, Cutts TA, McKinney J, Gerba CP. Predicted and measured virucidal efficacies of microbicides for emerging and reemerging viruses associated with WHO priority diseases. In: Disinfection of Viruses. Intech Open, London, UK. 2022; DOI: 10.5772/intechopen.102365

[21] World Health Organization. Prioritizing Diseases for Research and Development in Emergency Contexts. 2021;https://www.who.int/activities/prioritizing-diseases-for-research-and-development-in-emergency-contexts

[22] Zhou SS. Variability and relative order of susceptibility of non-enveloped viruses to chemical inactivation. In: Disinfection of Viruses. Intech Open, London, UK. 2022. DOI: 10.5772/intechopen.102727

[23] Nims RW, Plavsic M. Physical inactivation of SARS-CoV-2 and other coronaviruses: A review. In: Disinfection of Viruses. Intech Open, London, UK. 2022. DOI: 10.5772/intechopen.103161

[24] Ranjan K. Environmental persistence of SARS-CoV-2 and disinfection of worksurfaces in view of pandemic outbreak of COVID-19. In: Disinfection of Viruses. Intech Open, London, UK. 2022.

Section 1

Microbicides for Viral Inactivation

Chapter 1

Silver Ion (Ag^+) Formulations with Virucidal Efficacy against Severe Acute Respiratory Syndrome Coronavirus 2 (SARS-CoV-2)

Yutaka Nishihara, Hideo Eguchi and Sifang Steve Zhou

Abstract

This chapter focuses on viral efficacy evaluations of silver ion (Ag^+) formulations against severe acute respiratory syndrome coronavirus 2 (SARS-CoV-2), the virus associated with the COVID-19 pandemic and feline calicivirus (FCV), a surrogate for human norovirus. The chapter discusses the proposed mechanism of inactivation, with reference to some previously published articles. In addition, it discusses the background/current trend/future view of Ag^+ products that have been used widely as surface/environment disinfectants in daily life all over the world. In efficacy studies performed by using the standardized ASTM E1052 methodology, it was found that Ag^+ formulated with a low concentration (26% w/w) of ethanol displayed virucidal activity against SARS-CoV-2 and FeCV. These formulations might be useful for preventing the transmission of such viruses and limiting the outbreaks of emerging infectious diseases caused by coronaviruses and caliciviruses. To our knowledge, this is the first report describing the virucidal efficacy of an Ag^+ formulation, evaluated by using the standardized ASTM E1052 methodology, for inactivating SARS-CoV-2. Some characteristics of Ag^+-based virucides are discussed in this research report/minireview.

Keywords: COVID-19, feline calicivirus, liquid inactivation, SARS-CoV-2, silver ion (Ag^+), virucidal efficacy evaluation

1. Introduction

For over 6000 years and prior to the introduction of penicillin in the early 1940s, silver has been the main antimicrobial used by mankind [1]. Few people today are aware that, by 1940 prior to the introduction of penicillin, in the USA alone more than 50 silver-based antimicrobial products had been marketed in different formulations (solutions, ointments, colloids, or foils) for topical, oral, and intramuscular injections [2]. In brief, between 1900 and 1940, tens of thousands of patients were treated with colloidal silver, with several million doses of silver administered intravenously [1]. Since the early 2000s, antibiotic resistance of microbes has been of increasing concern. For both antiviral and antimicrobial applications, silver ion (Ag^+)- and silver nanoparticle (AgNP)-based formulations have displayed an advantage in this respect, attacking bacteria and viruses in multiple ways and thereby limiting the chances of both viruses and bacteria to develop resistance to such formulations [2, 3].

This chapter describes the virucidal efficacy of a silver ion formulation, evaluated by using the standardized ASTM International (ASTM) E1052 methodology [4], for inactivating severe acute respiratory syndrome coronavirus 2 (SARS-CoV-2) and feline calicivirus (FeCV). The chapter also includes a discussion of the proposed mechanism of inactivation, with reference to some previously published articles. Some characteristics of Ag^+- and AGNP-based virucides also are discussed in this research report/minireview.

2. Rediscovery of the antimicrobial potential of silver ion (Ag^+) and AgNP

The discovery that the antibacterial activity of AgNP is chiefly due to Ag^+ nonetheless led Xiu et al. [5] to recommend the use of AgNP in antimicrobial formulations because AgNP are less prone than Ag^+ to binding and sequestering by naturally occurring ligands. For this reason, it was thought that AgNP might better deliver Ag^+ to the bacterial cytoplasm via the acidic cell membrane.

The rediscovery of silver as a powerful and broad-spectrum antimicrobial since the early 2000s has several lessons to teach us. The demonstration of the efficacy of silver, this time in the form of AgNP, against drug-resistant bacteria such as Pseudomonas aeruginosa, ampicillin-resistant Escherichia coli, erythromycin-resistant Streptococcus pyogenes, and methicillin-resistant Staphylococcus aureus (MRSA) is encouraging, in view of the continuous increase in multidrug-resistant human pathogenic microbes [6]. Research advances suggesting new medical uses of silver, including nanocrystalline silver, have been rapid and numerous products have been marketed, especially for healing wounds. The rediscovery of the medical uses of silver provides a noticeable example of the interface of chemistry and medicine in enhancing the real (and nonlinear) progress of scientific research.

The use of AgNP for various biological and biomedical applications, such as antibacterial, antifungal, antiviral, anti-inflammatory, anticancer, and anti-angiogenic has now been described [7]. Under these circumstances, there have not been many efficacy studies for Ag^+ compared to AgNP. In our development work, we have conducted a series of virucidal tests of Ag^+ formulations against SARS-CoV-2 and FeCV. These are enveloped and non-enveloped viruses, respectively, which are human pathogens or surrogate viruses for human pathogens that continue to impact health. Additional virucidal agents with broad-spectrum efficacy might be useful for infection prevention and control (IPAC) during the present or future viral epidemics/pandemics.

3. Virucidal efficacy evaluation of Ag^+ formulations against SARS-CoV-2 and FeCV

3.1 Materials and methods

1. Challenge viruses

    - Severe acute respiratory syndrome coronavirus 2 (SARS-CoV-2): Isolate USA-WA1/2020, BEI Resources, NR-1586.

- Feline calicivirus (FeCV): ATCC VR-782 (used as a surrogate for human norovirus).

2. Host (detector) cells

    - For SARS-CoV-2: Vero E6 cells (African green monkey kidney); ATCC CRL-1586, grown in minimal essential medium (MEM) containing 5% fetal bovine serum (FBS).

    - For FeCV: CrFK cells (Crandell-Rees Feline Kidney); ATCC CCL-94, grown in RPMI 1640 medium containing 5% FBS.

3. Test formulations

    - 5 ppm Ag^+ solution in water; pH 6.1.

    - 5 ppm Ag^+ solution in water containing 26% w/w ethanol, pH 4.2.

4. Synopsis of the ASTM E1052 testing methodology (Suspension Time-Kill Test for Virus) [4]

    - Each stock challenge virus had a titer of $\geq 6 \log_{10}$ infectious units/mL, in a culture medium containing 5% fetal bovine serum as the organic soil challenge.

    - The test product was prepared for the use-dilution and an equal volume of the dilution medium (minimum essential medium containing 2% newborn calf serum) was prepared to serve a virus control.

    - The prepared viral inoculum was added to the test formulation and the virus recovery control at a ratio of virus (one part) + test formulation or dilution medium (nine parts).

    - Upon completion of the contact time, the test and recovery suspensions were neutralized by dilution into a chemical neutralizer (minimum essential medium +10% newborn calf serum +0.5% lecithin +1 mM EDTA).

    - For the cytotoxicity control, an aliquot of the use-dilution of the test formulation was mixed with the dilution medium (in lieu of the virus) and then neutralized in an identical manner to the test suspension.

    - For the neutralization control, an aliquot of the use-dilution of the test formulation was mixed with the dilution medium, neutralized, and then spiked with a low level of virus.

    - The neutralized test suspension, virus recovery control, cytotoxicity control, and neutralization control suspensions were serially diluted in the dilution medium. Each diluted solution was plated in quadruplicate to host cell monolayers in a 24-well plate. Maintenance medium was then added to each well, and the host cells with the inoculated virus were allowed to incubate for 4–9 days at 37°C with 5% CO_2.

- Infectivity assay: The residual infectious virus in both test and control conditions was determined by viral-induced cytopathic effect (CPE) that was observed by light microscopy. Cytotoxicity control wells were examined for cytotoxicity to host cells caused by the test formulation. The resulting virus-specific CPE and test formulation-specific cytotoxic effects were scored by examining both test and control cultures.

- Determination of efficacy (calculation): The virus titers in 50% tissue culture infectious doses per mL ($TCID_{50}$/mL) were determined by using the method of Spearman-Kärber [8] and the amounts of infectious virus present prior to and after treatment were quantified as shown below.

  The virus load was calculated according to Eq. (1):

$$\text{Virus Load } (\text{Log}_{10}\ \text{TCID}_{50}) = \text{Virus Titer } (\text{Log}_{10}\ \text{TCID}_{50}/\text{mL}) + \text{Log}_{10}\ [\text{Volume (mL)} \times \text{Volume correction } (\textit{e.g.}, \text{neutralization})] \tag{1}$$

The Log_{10} Inactivation was calculated according to Eq. (2):

$$\text{Log}_{10}\ \text{Inactivation} = \text{Virus Recovery Control } (\text{Log}_{10}\ \text{TCID}_{50}) - \text{Test } (\text{Log}_{10}\ \text{TCID}_{50}) \tag{2}$$

5. Virucidal test acceptance criteria [4]

- Viral-induced CPE must be distinguishable from the microbicide-induced cytotoxic effects (if any).

- Viruses must be recovered from the neutralizer effectiveness/virus interference control (not exhibiting cytotoxicity).

- The cell viability control (assay negative control) must not exhibit viral CPE.

Challenge virus	Log_{10} inactivation (log_{10} reduction in titer)		After contact time
	5 ppm Ag^+ solution	5 ppm Ag^+ + 26% (w/w) ethanol	(minutes)
Enveloped virus			
Severe acute respiratory syndrome coronavirus 2 (SARS-CoV-2; *Coronaviridae*)	0.70	≥3.72	1
	3.05	NT	360
Non-enveloped virus			
Feline calicivirus (FeCV; *Caliciviridae*)	NT	0.70	1
	NT	≥4.30	30

Ag^+ = silver ion; NT = not tested; ppm = parts per million.

Table 1.
Virucidal efficacy of Ag^+ formulations against SARS-CoV-2 and FeCV evaluated in suspension inactivation studies.

3.2 Results of inactivation studies

Virucidal activity studies were conducted according to a standardized quantitative suspension testing method ASTM E1052–20 [4]. Evaluation of virucidal activity against the enveloped coronavirus, SARS-CoV-2, demonstrated that 5 ppm Ag^+ formulated without ethanol caused minimal (<1 $\log_{10}$) inactivation within 1-min contact time, but 3.1 $\log_{10}$ inactivations after 360 minutes (6 h) (**Table 1**). On the other hand, 5 ppm Ag^+ formulated with a low (26% w/w) concentration of alcohol caused ≥3.72 $\log_{10}$ inactivations of SARS-CoV-2 within 1-min contact time (**Table 1**).

The 5 ppm Ag^+ formulated with 26% w/w ethanol also demonstrated efficacy (≥ 4.3 $\log_{10}$ inactivations) against the non-enveloped calicivirus, FeCV, within 30-min contact time, but only minimal (<1 $\log_{10}$) inactivation of FeCV within 1-min contact time (**Table 1**).

4. Silver ion (Ag^+) mechanisms of microbicidal activity

The broad antimicrobial activity of silver nanoparticles (AgNP) includes efficacy against over 650 microorganisms, including bacteria, fungi, and viruses. This activity is primarily due to the leaching of Ag^+ ions from the outer surface of the AgNP [9]. Xiu et al. [10] demonstrated that anaerobic conditions (i.e., in the absence of oxygen) prevent the Ag^0 oxidation and Ag^+ leaching from AgNP that is favored in acidic environments [Eqs. (3) and (4)].

$$4\,\mathrm{Ag}^0 + O_2 \rightarrow 2\,\mathrm{Ag}_2O \tag{3}$$

$$2\,\mathrm{Ag}_2O + 4\,H^+ \rightarrow 4\,\mathrm{Ag}^+ + 2\,H_2O \tag{4}$$

Under anaerobic conditions, AgNP has no detectable effects on E. coli at concentrations 7665 times higher than the minimum lethal concentration of Ag^+ (0.025 mg/L) under the same exposure conditions. In addition, these authors found that the minimum lethal concentration for AgNP under anaerobic conditions was thousands of times higher than the minimum lethal concentration observed under aerobic conditions [10]. This discovery led the researchers to conclude that the antibacterial activity could be controlled by modulating the Ag^+ release (leaching) kinetics through modifications to the AgNP size, shape, and surface characteristics, including the presence of a coating [10].

There are four known antimicrobial actions of AgNP [11, 12]: 1) adhesion to the microbial cell membrane; 2) penetration of AgNP into the cell, causing disruption of biomolecules and intracellular damage; 3) induction of cellular toxicity mediated by reactive oxygen species (ROS), resulting in oxidative stress to the cell; and 4) disruption of signal transduction pathways of the cells.

When microbes are exposed to AgNP, the nanoparticles tend to stick or adhere to the cell wall or membrane due to the electrostatic attraction between the positive charge of Ag^+ generated during oxidation of AgNP and the negatively charged cell membrane of microorganisms (**Figure 1**). AgNP also displays a strong affinity for the sulfur-containing proteins in the microbial cell wall. The attachment of AgNP to the cell membrane causes irreversible morphological changes in the membrane structure. This can also cause a loss in the integrity of the lipid bilayer and changes in the permeability of the cell membrane. Alterations in such structures can cause increased permeability of the cell membrane, which, in turn, impacts the ability of the cell to regulate essential activities. For instance, the binding of AgNP and subsequent leaching of Ag^+ can alter transport and release of potassium ion (K^+),

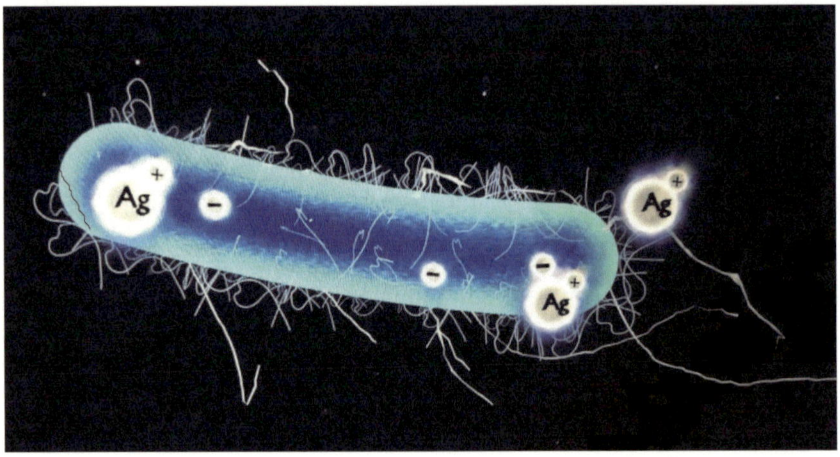

Figure 1.
Schematic depiction of interaction of extracellular Ag^+ with the bacterial cell membrane and subsequent entry of Ag^+ into the cell. Ag^+ and AgNP enter the bacterial cell membrane by porin proteins. Within the bacterial cell membrane, Ag^+ causes the formation of several highly oxidizing species, such as hydroxyl and superoxide free-radicals and hydrogen peroxide (H_2O_2), which quickly oxidizes DNA and RNA, and denature proteins. This results in cell membrane rupture and pore formation. Leakage of intracellular contents and cell lysis results [3].

thus affecting the transport activity of cells. An increase in cell membrane permeability may also cause loss or leakage of cellular contents such as cytoplasmic proteins, ions, and cellular energy reservoirs (adenosine triphosphate; ATP).

Following the adhesion of AgNP to the microbial membrane, the nanoparticles can penetrate the cell and impact important biomolecules and cellular activities. AgNP is able to enter Gram-negative bacteria, such as E. coli, through water-filled channels in the membrane called porins. After penetration of AgNP into the cells, these nanoparticles will start to bind with cellular structures and biomolecules, such as proteins, lipids, and DNA, thus damaging the internal structure of the bacteria. Any leached Ag^+ binds to negatively charged proteins, altering the proteins structurally and eventually resulting in denaturing of the proteins.

Another mechanism of action of AgNP is the production of ROS, which causes cellular oxidative stress in microbes. Reactive oxygen species is a general term for oxygenated compounds that are involved in various cellular biological events. These can include but are not limited to superoxide, hydrogen peroxide, and hydroxyl radicals. The antibacterial potential of AgNP is usually related to the ability of the nanoparticles to produce ROS and increase the oxidative stress in the cells. Production of intercellular ROS is thought to be the most important indicator of toxicity related to AgNP, as the ROS may induce lipid damage and leakage of cellular biomolecules, and may eventually lead to cell apoptosis [11, 12].

The virucidal efficacy of Ag^+ and AgNP is mediated by the following types of interactions: 1) the Ag^+/AgNP bind to spike proteins of enveloped viruses, inhibiting the attachment of these viruses to host cell receptors (**Figure 2**); and 2) Ag^+/AgNP bind to the genomic DNA or RNA of both enveloped and non-enveloped viruses, inhibiting the replication or propagation of the virus inside the host cells.

For example, in the case of the human immunodeficiency virus (HIV-1; family *Retroviridae*, enveloped), the AgNP binds to the sulfur groups of gp120 protein spikes on the viral envelope, thereby preventing infectivity due to the fusion of the viral envelope with the host cell membrane [13]. Similarly, the attachment and entry of herpes simplex virus type 1 (HSV-1; family *Herpesviridae*, enveloped) into cells involve interaction between viral envelope glycoproteins and cell surface heparan sulfate (HS). Viral entry can be prevented by AgNP capped with mercaptoethane sulfonate

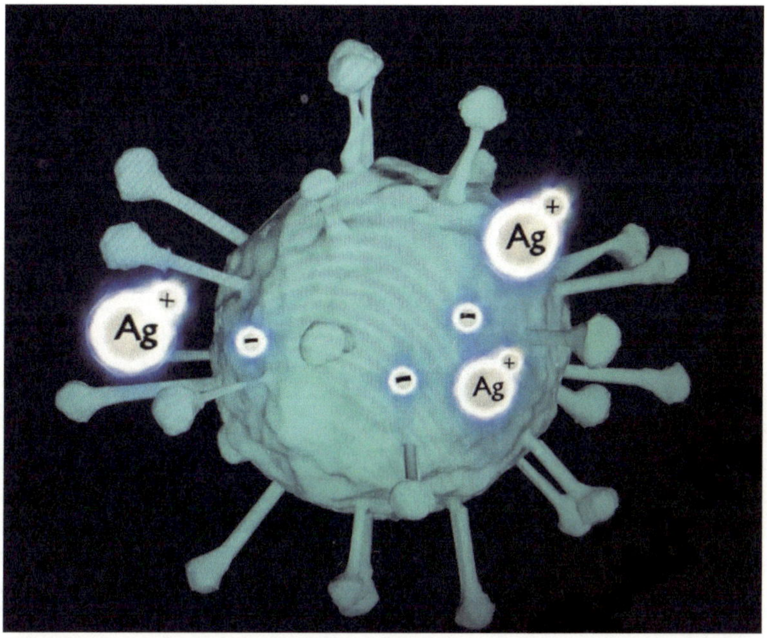

Figure 2.
Schematic depiction of interaction of extracellular Ag^+ with enveloped viruses, such as SARS-CoV-2.

targeting the virus and competing for its binding to cellular HS through their sulfonate end groups [14]. The antiviral mechanism of inorganic metals such as copper and silver against influenza A viruses appears to be mediated through the inactivation of hemagglutinin (HA) and neuraminidase (NA) cell surface proteins [15].

It was demonstrated in experimental RSV infection studies by Morris et al. [16] that AgNP caused a reduction in RSV. In the mouse model, the antiviral activity appeared to be mediated to a large extent by neutrophils, which were recruited in higher numbers to the airways and activated *via* a neutrophil-specific program of cytokines. This was reported as the first *in vivo* study demonstrating antiviral activity of AgNP during RSV infection.

5. Discussion

Silver ion (Ag^+) has been used since ancient times for various purposes [1]. Silver plays a certain role in mythology and has found various usages as a metaphor. In folklore, silver was commonly thought to have mystic powers. For example, a bullet cast from silver was supposed in such folklore to be the only weapon effective against a werewolf, witch, or other monsters. From this mythology, the idiom of the silver bullet resulted in figuratively referring to any simple solution with very high effectiveness or almost miraculous results, as in the widely discussed software engineering paper "No Silver Bullet" [17]. Other mythic powers attributed to silver have included detection of poisons and facilitation of passage into the mythical realm of the fairies.

In medicine, silver has been incorporated into wound dressings and used as an antibiotic coating in medical devices. Wound dressings containing silver sulfadiazine or silver nanoparticles have been used to treat external infections. Silver has also been used in urinary catheters for reducing catheter-related urinary tract infections and in endotracheal breathing tubes for reducing ventilator-associated pneumonia [18, 19]. Silver ion is bioactive and, at sufficient concentration, readily kills bacteria *in vitro*. Silver and silver nanoparticles are used as antimicrobial ingredients in a variety of industrial, health care, and domestic applications. For example, infusing clothing with AgNP allows the items to remain odorless longer [20].

Silver ion (Ag^+) displays broad-spectrum antimicrobial action, with efficacy against various bacteria, fungi, and viruses. Due to their versatility, AgNP is currently used as microbicides in wound dressings, medical devices, deodorant sprays, and fabrics. Studies have demonstrated the virucidal efficacy of AgNP against human pathogenic viruses, including enveloped viruses such as respiratory syncytial virus (RSV), influenza virus, hepatitis B virus (HBV), and human immunodeficiency virus (HIV), as well as non-enveloped viruses such as human norovirus [2]. In addition, Ag^+ has been shown to possess virucidal efficacy against severe acute respiratory syndrome coronavirus (SARS-CoV) [21] and SARS-CoV-2 [22, 23]. AgNP formulations have been proposed for cleaning inanimate surfaces to efficiently control the ongoing COVID-19 pandemic [23]. The hypothesis was based on the proposed mechanism of action of AgNP, involving binding to the spike glycoprotein of the virus, thereby inhibiting the binding of the virus to the host cells. Dissemination of respiratory pathogens such as SARS-CoV-2 from infected to susceptible individuals is believed to occur directly, *via* respiratory droplets and droplet nuclei/aerosols, and indirectly, through contaminated high-touch environmental surfaces (HITES) [24]. SARS-CoV-2 has been reported to remain infectious on contaminated HITES for hours to days [25–27].

The Ag^+ formulations discussed in this chapter are not considered silver zeolites or silver zirconium phosphate. These Ag^+ formulations are, therefore, not in scope for the European Union ban on the use of certain silver compounds in antimicrobial products [28].

Until the virucidal efficacy of microbicides is empirically demonstrated for SARS-CoV-2 specifically, the EPA has allowed agents to be used on the basis of their activity against other enveloped and non-enveloped viruses (**Box 1**). Virucidal efficacy of a selection of formulated microbicidal actives against SARS-CoV-2 has, to date, been assumed based on efficacy data obtained using other coronaviruses, or based on non-standardized methods of assessing viral inactivation (i.e., $\log_{10}$ reduction in infectious titer) in suspension without details of the testing method used, including use of appropriate controls. To date, only limited virucidal testing against SARS-CoV-2 has been demonstrated definitively through testing conducted per standardized surface and suspension methodologies [27].

> On March 5, 2020, the US Environmental Protection Agency (EPA) announced the release of a new list [29] of EPA-registered disinfectant products that were considered as qualified for use against SARS-CoV-2, the coronavirus that causes the disease COVID-19. Products on EPA's "List N: Disinfectants for Use Against SARS-CoV-2" are registered disinfectants qualified for use against SARS-CoV-2 through EPA's Emerging Viral Pathogen Program (EVPP) [30]. Currently, there are 85 products listed that are qualified for use against SARS-CoV-2. Of note, EPA states that if the directions for use for viruses/virucidal activity of the listed products provide different contact times or dilutions, the longest contact time or most concentrated solution should be used. The EPA initially issued guidance for the EVPP in 2016; the program was intended to "expedite the process for registrants to provide useful information to the public" regarding products that should be effective against emerging viral pathogens.
>
> According to the EVPP, in the event of an outbreak, companies with pre-approved products can make off-label claims (e.g., technical literature distributed exclusively to healthcare facilities, physicians, nurses, and public health officials; 1–800 consumer information services; company websites (non-label related); and social media) for use of these products against the outbreak virus. These emerging pathogen statements do not appear on marketed (final print) product labels. Products that meet EPA's criteria for use against SARS-CoV-2 can be searched using the EPA database [29]. This database allows users to search by criteria such as EPA registration number, the active ingredient, use site, surface types, contact time, and keywords.

Box 1.
EPA-registered disinfectant products qualified for use against SARS-CoV-2.

6. Conclusions

In order to expand the known set of virucidal agents with efficacy for SARS-CoV-2, we conducted virucidal efficacy studies on Ag^+ with and without 26% (w/w) ethanol, according to the ASTM E1052 standardized suspension methodology [4]. The Ag^+ formulation with low concentrations of ethanol should be less flammable than 70% ethanol at the time of use or at the time of storage and during shipping. The formulation without ethanol proved effective for the enveloped SARS-CoV-2 virus, while efficacy for non-enveloped viruses such as FeCV required formulation with 26% ethanol.

To our knowledge, this is the first report of the virucidal efficacy of Ag^+ formulations, evaluated using standardized ASTM methodology, for inactivating SARS-CoV-2. From the viewpoint of infection prevention and control, effective surface disinfectants such as the Ag^+ ion formulations discussed in this chapter represent a possible intervention for interrupting the transmission of SARS-CoV-2.

Acknowledgements

The authors would like to thank Dr. Raymond Nims for his assistance during the writing process.

Conflict of interest

The authors declare no conflict of interest.

Author details

Yutaka Nishihara[1]*, Hideo Eguchi[2] and Sifang Steve Zhou[3]

1 Bizen Chemical Co., Ltd., Okayama-City, Okayama, Japan

2 Sun Techno Co., Ltd., Obu-City, Aichi, Japan

3 Microbac Laboratories, Sterling, Virginia, USA

*Address all correspondence to: hndragon555@gmail.com

References

[1] Alexander JW. History of the medical use of silver. Surgical Infections. 2009; **10**:289-292

[2] Galdiero S, Falanga A, Vitiello M, Cantisani M, Marra V, Galdiero M. Silver nanoparticles as potential antiviral agents. Molecules. 2011;**16**(10): 8894-8918

[3] Gugala N, Lemire J, Chatfield-Reed K, Yan Y, Chua G, Turner RJ. Using a chemical genetic screen to enhance our understanding of the antibacterial properties of silver. Genes. 2018;**9**(7): 344. DOI: 10.3390/genes9070344

[4] ASTM International. ASTM E1052-20. Standard practice to assess the activity of microbicides against viruses in suspension. 2020. DOI: 10.1520/E1052-20 https://www.astm.org/Standards/E1052.htm

[5] Xiu Z-M, Ma J, Alvarez PJJ. Differential effect of common ligands and molecular oxygen on antimicrobial activity of silver nanoparticles versus silver ions. Environmental Science & Technology. 2011;**45**(20):9003-9008

[6] Rai MK, Deshmukh SD, Ingle AP, Gade AK. Silver nanoparticles: the powerful nanoweapon against multidrug-resistant bacteria. Journal of Applied Microbiology. 2012;**112**(5):841-852

[7] Zhang X-F, Liu Z-G, Shen W, Gurunathan S. Silver nanoparticles: synthesis, characterization, properties, applications, and therapeutic approaches. International Journal of Molecular Sciences. 2016;**17**(9):1534. DOI: 10.3390/ijms17091534

[8] Kärber G. Beitrag zur kollektiven Behandlung pharmakologischer Reihenversuche. Naunyn-Schmiedebergs Archiv für Experimentelle Pathologie und Pharmakologie. 1931;**162**:480-483

[9] Dakal TC, Kumar A, Majumdar RS, Yadav V. Mechanistic basis of antimicrobial actions of silver nanoparticles. Frontiers in Microbiology. 2016;**7**:1831. DOI: 10.3389/fmicb.2016.01831

[10] Xiu Z-M, Q-b Z, Puppala HL, Colvin VL, Alvarez PJJ. Negligible particle-specific antibacterial activity of silver nanoparticles. Nano Letters. 2012; **12**(8):4271-4275

[11] Salleh A, Naomi R, Utami ND, Mohammad AW, Mahmoudi E, Mustafa N, et al. The potential of silver nanoparticles for antiviral and antibacterial applications: a mechanism of action. Nanomaterials. 2020;**10**(8): 1566. DOI: 10.3390/nano10081566

[12] Yin IX, Zhang J, Zhao IS, Mei ML, Chu CH. The antibacterial mechanism of silver nanoparticles and its application in dentistry. International Journal of Nanomedicine. 2020;**15**:2555-2562

[13] Lara HH, Ayala-Nuñez NV, Ixtepan-Turrent L, Rodriguez-Padilla C. Mode of antiviral action of silver nanoparticles against HIV-1. Journal of Nanobiotechnology. 2010;**8**:1. DOI: 10.1186/1477-3155-8-1

[14] Baram-Pinto D, Shukla S, Perkas N, Gedanken A, Sarid R. Inhibition of herpes simplex virus type 1 infection by silver nanoparticles capped with mercaptoethane sulfonate. Bioconjugate Chemistry. 2009;**20**(8):1497-1502

[15] Minoshima M, Lu Y, Kimura T, Nakano R, Ishiguro H, Kubota Y, et al. Comparison of the antiviral effect of solid-state copper and silver compounds. Journal of Hazardous Materials. 2016;**312**: 1-7. DOI: 10.1016/j.jhazmat.2016.03.023

[16] Morris D, Ansar M, Speshock J, Ivanciuc T, Qu Y, Casola A, et al. Antiviral and immunomodulatory

activity of silver nanoparticles in experimental RSV infection. Viruses. 2019;**11**(8):732. DOI: 10.3390/v11080732

[17] Raymond ES. The Cathedral and the Bazaar 1997: "No Silver Bullet" paper.

[18] Beattie M, Taylor J. Silver alloy vs. uncoated urinary catheters: a systematic review of the literature. Journal of Clinical Nursing. 2011;**20**(15–16): 2098-2108

[19] Bouadma L, Wolff M, Lucet J-C. Ventilator-associated pneumonia and its prevention. Current Opinion in Infectious Diseases. 2012;**25**(4):395-404

[20] Maillard J-Y, Hartemann P. Silver as an antimicrobial: facts and gaps in knowledge. Critical Reviews in Microbiology. 2012;**39**(4):373-383

[21] Han J, Chen L, Duan S-M, Yang Q-X, Yang M, Gao C, et al. Efficient and quick inactivation of SARS coronavirus and other microbes exposed to the surfaces of some metal catalysts. Biomedical and Environmental Sciences. 2005;**18**(3):176-180

[22] Talebian S, Wallace GG, Schroeder A, Stellacci F, Conde J. Nanotechnology-based disinfectants and sensors for SARS-CoV-2. Nature Nanotechnology. 2020;**15**:618-621

[23] Jeremiah SS, Miyakawa K, Morita T, Yamaoka Y, Ryo A. Potent antiviral effect of silver nanoparticles on SARS-CoV-2. Biochemical and Biophysical Research Communications. 2020; **533**(1):195-200. https://doi.org/10.1016/j.bbrc.2020.09.018

[24] Ijaz MK, Nims RW, McKinney J. Indirect transmission of severe acute respiratory syndrome coronavirus virus 2 (SARS-CoV-2) infection; what do we know and what don't we know? Journal of Infection Control and Hospital Epidemiology. 2021;Feb 9:1-2. DOI: 10.1017/ice.2021.57

[25] World Health Organization. Modes of transmission of virus causing COVID-19: implications for IPC precaution recommendations. 2020; Available at: https://www.who.int/news-room/commentaries/detail/modes-of-transmission-of-viruscausing-covid-19-implications-for-ipc-precaution-recommendations.

[26] AWH C, JTS C, MRA P, KPY H, Yen H-L, MCW C, et al. Stability of SARS-CoV-2 in different environmental conditions. The Lancet Microbe. May 2020;**1**(1):e10. https://doi.org/10.1016/S2666-5247(20)30003-3

[27] Ijaz MK, Nims RW, Zhou SS, Whitehead K, Srinivasan V, Kapes T, et al. Microbicidal actives with virucidal efficacy against SARS-CoV-2 and other beta- and alpha-coronaviruses and implications for future emerging coronaviruses and other enveloped viruses. Scientific Reports. 2021;**11**:5626 https://doi.org/10.1038/s41598-021-84842-1

[28] European Chemicals Agency. Biocidal Products Committee proposes not to approve three silver-containing active substances. 2018; ECHA/NR/18/59: https://echa.europa.eu/-/biocidal-products-committee-proposes-not-to-approve-three-silver-containing-active-substances

[29] Environmental Protection Agency. EPA Registered Disinfectants. available at: https://pgpro.com/en-us/whats-new/epa-registered-cleaning-products/?gclid=Cj0KCQjw6NmHBhD2ARIsAI3hrM2uqIoAVAi7stVRAPoaxjnXTLAJM7y0SKTArCJJ3yi179yGD5DO4M4aAk_mEALw_wcB

[30] Environmental Protection Agency. Emerging Viral Pathogen Guidance for Antimicrobial Pesticides. https://www.epa.gov/pesticide-registration/emerging-viral-pathogen-guidance-antimicrobial-pesticides

Chapter 2

Dry Hydrogen Peroxide for Viral Inactivation

Chris Lee and John R. Henneman

Abstract

Hydrogen peroxide is a common antiseptic and disinfectant that is effective against both enveloped and non-enveloped viruses, and it is sometimes used as a fumigant to achieve disinfection of indoor spaces. While it is effective as a fumigant, it cannot be used continuously, allowing for possible recontamination of the treated spaces between applications. A novel method of hydrogen peroxide application, termed "Dry Hydrogen Peroxide" (DHP™), generates molecules of hydrogen peroxide in a true gas state at concentrations low enough to be used continuously within spaces occupied by humans. This chapter explores the efficacy of DHP against a variety of viruses, both enveloped and non-enveloped. On surfaces, DHP achieved a ≥ 99.8% reduction (≥2.62 log_{10} inactivation) of infectious H1N1 influenza A (enveloped) compared to the control condition within 1 hour, and it achieved a 99.8% reduction (2.62 log_{10} inactivation) of infectious feline calicivirus (non-enveloped) compared to the control condition within 6 hours. DHP also achieved a 99.8% reduction 2.62 log_{10} inactivation) of airborne MS2 bacteriophage (non-enveloped) within 1 hour in comparison to the control condition. These inactivation efficacy results, combined with results from recent clinical studies, indicate that DHP represents an effective adjunct technology that can mitigate viral load between intermittent applications of other types of disinfectants.

Keywords: viral inactivation, dry hydrogen peroxide, disinfectant, hydroxyl radical, biocidal action

1. Introduction

Since the late 19th century, hydrogen peroxide (H_2O_2) has been used as a disinfectant and antiseptic due to its potent antimicrobial properties against a wide range of pathogens [1]. Hydrogen peroxide attacks the essential external structures of pathogens (i.e. cell walls, viral envelopes, etc.) via a simple oxidation reaction, thereby weakening the pathogen's physical structure until it ultimately lyses from its own osmotic pressure [2–4]. Most commonly, H_2O_2 is used as a liquid antiseptic and disinfectant, but solutions of H_2O_2 are also vaporized and dispersed as a method of disinfection of indoor spaces. This process, however, requires the complete evacuation of personnel from the treated spaces, both during and for some time after the treatment, to protect human occupants from the toxic effects of the highly concentrated droplets [5, 6]. Symptoms of overexposure to H_2O_2 include irritation of the eyes, nose, throat, skin, and/or lungs, and concentrations over 75 parts per million (ppm) are considered "immediately dangerous to life or health" in humans [7, 8]. Droplets of vaporized hydrogen peroxide, depending on the generator, may contain concentrations of approximately 400 ppm [9], therefore, while vaporized hydrogen peroxide is extremely effective as a sterilant, its potential for use in continuously occupied spaces is limited by its potency and potential toxicity to human occupants [10, 11].

Hydrogen peroxide is also an essential component of the human respiratory system, with human lungs maintaining an equilibrium concentration between 10^{-6} and 10^{-4} M via the lactoperoxidase system of enzymes [12]. Two enzymes within this system, known as the Duox compound, constantly produce hydrogen peroxide, while the third enzyme, lactoperoxidase, converts that hydrogen peroxide into an even stronger oxidizing agent, the hypothiocyanite ion ($OSCN^-$) [12, 13]. This enzymatic system allows the human body to tolerate low levels of hydrogen peroxide exposure without experiencing irritation or damage.

Recently, a new method of hydrogen peroxide generation and delivery termed Dry Hydrogen Peroxide (DHP™) was developed, with the goal of enabling safe continuous microbial inactivation to occur in occupied indoor spaces either when installed within an existing HVAC system or as a stand-alone device (**Figures 1** and **2**) [14]. DHP is produced by devices that include a 363 nm wavelength ultraviolet A (UV-A) bulb, which activates a proprietary photocatalyst that has been applied to a two-dimensional framed polyester mesh, referred to as a "sail". Photons of UV-A radiation from the bulb excite electrons in the catalyst, promoting them to a higher energy state. This creates a positively charged "electron hole" in the valence band in the catalyst atoms, creating an active site. When ambient humidity (H_2O) is adsorbed into these active sites, an electron is scavenged from the water molecule. This causes a subsequent release of a proton (H^+) by the water molecule, and the resulting structure is a hydroxyl radical ($OH^{\cdot}$). The catalyst now has a free electron, a proton (H^+), and a hydroxyl radical available to perform oxidation reactions. Under normal circumstances, these three components simply combine to produce a water molecule in the gas phase. DHP technology, however, uses a proprietary plasma separation process to isolate hydroxyl radicals from the subatomic particles. This separation of the plasma allows for the hydroxyl radicals to combine and form stable molecules of hydrogen peroxide in a pure gas state (DHP), which are then dispersed throughout the space being treated. The subatomic particles that remain on the catalyst are then scavenged by ambient diatomic oxygen (O_2), forming more molecules of DHP by means of reduction. The concentrations of DHP that are produced through this process are well below the OSHA safety limit of 1 ppm, allowing the lactoperoxidase system to easily maintain the equilibrium concentration of hydrogen peroxide to the level naturally present in the lungs [12, 13]. Additionally,

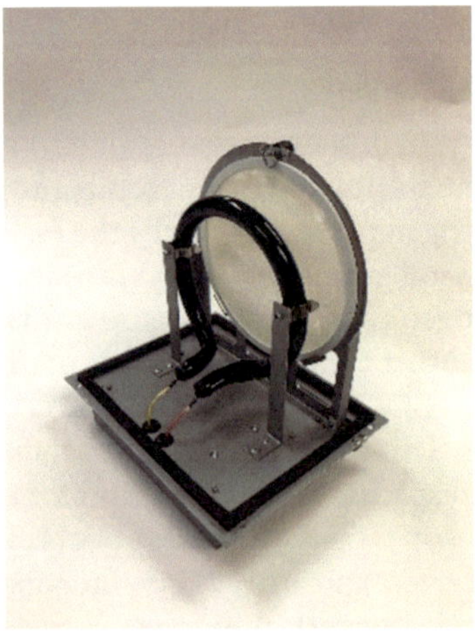

Figure 1.
In-line Dry Hydrogen peroxide (DHP) device intended for use in an HVAC system.

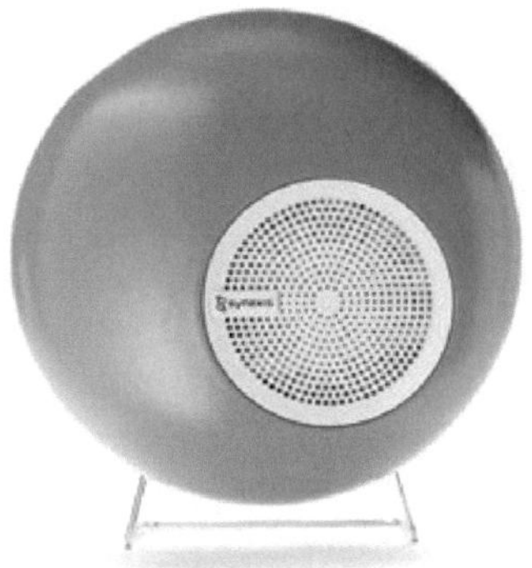

Figure 2.
Stand-alone Dry Hydrogen Peroxide (DHP) device.

it has been confirmed that DHP devices produced by the patent holder do not produce ozone, according to Underwriter's Laboratories (UL) Standards 867 and 2998 [15, 16]. A recent study performed by Ramirez et al. reported no incidence of symptoms associated with hydrogen peroxide overexposure in pediatric oncology patients who were continuously exposed to DHP during their stay in a Pediatric Intensive Care Unit (PICU) [17].

Due to the novelty and mechanism of generation of DHP, this disinfection system is often confused with older technologies, such as vaporized hydrogen peroxide, bipolar ionization, and photocatalytic oxidation, though it is distinct from each of those technologies.

2. Dry hydrogen peroxide and vaporized hydrogen peroxide

While DHP and vaporized hydrogen peroxide both utilize hydrogen peroxide to reduce infectious pathogen burdens in a treated indoor space, there are several notable differences between the two technologies. The most apparent difference between DHP and vaporized hydrogen peroxide is that DHP is a true gas composed of individual molecules exhibiting near ideal gas behavior [18], whereas VHP is an aerosol of highly concentrated aqueous droplets. As a result, vaporized hydrogen peroxide effectively sterilizes a room, but it also may lead to aerosol H_2O_2 concentrations which exceed the safety limits for human exposure. Vaporized hydrogen peroxide may only be used in vacated areas. Other precautionary measures, such as sealing doors, windows, and HVAC systems, must be taken before use as well, in order to prevent unintended dissemination of H_2O_2 to adjacent spaces [5, 6, 9–11]. Further, in aqueous form, hydrogen peroxide forms a weak acid which is corrosive to some materials, equipment, and furnishings. Dry Hydrogen Peroxide, on the other hand, is much less concentrated, and does not cause such material compatibility issues. Dry Hydrogen Peroxide can be applied for an unlimited time of exposure and can be used in spaces occupied by humans. Dry Hydrogen Peroxide therefore represents a highly effective adjunct to the intermittent usage of harsher disinfectants.

2.1 Dry hydrogen peroxide and bipolar ionization

Bipolar ionization creates a plasma consisting of positive ions, negative ions, and free radicals, with the intention of releasing them into a space. This plasma can be generated in multiple ways, but the two primary types of bipolar ionization are corona discharge and needlepoint. Both types of bipolar ionization utilize sets of oppositely charged electrodes to ionize ambient humidity and oxygen as the indoor air passes through the device. Corona discharge bipolar ionization is rarely utilized currently, due to the potential for generation of ozone; accordingly, most manufacturers have switched to needlepoint ionization [19]. Manufacturers of needlepoint bipolar ionization (NPBI) claim that the electrodes used in the devices produce an electric field with a voltage below 12 eV to eliminate the potential for ozone generation [20]. Dry Hydrogen Peroxide and bipolar ionization each utilize ambient humidity and oxygen in their generation processes and continuously disperse their products throughout treated spaces; however, DHP is produced as stable H_2O_2 molecules, while bipolar ions are an unstable plasma. Additionally, neutrally charged H_2O_2 generated from DHP can travel long distances, whereas the oppositely charged ions created by bipolar ionization may rapidly recombine, diminishing the effective concentration as distance from the device increases [21, 22].

2.2 Dry hydrogen peroxide and photocatalytic oxidation

Both DHP and Photocatalytic Oxidation (PCO) technologies utilize photocatalysis during their respective processes, however DHP devices are not PCO devices [18, 23]. DHP technology uses a plasma-separation process to specifically produce free H_2O_2. Photocatalytic Oxidation technology, however, rapidly consumes any H_2O_2 that may form in the plasma, because H_2O_2 has a highly positive reduction potential (0.71 eV) and will be immediately reduced to water by subatomic particles in the plasma [24]. Photocatalytic Oxidation devices rely on a dense internal plasma zone within the device, but the microbicidal properties of the plasma only affect airborne microbes that circulate through the device, unless the device also produces ozone, which would impact microbes outside of the device.

2.3 Efficacy of DHP for inactivating viruses

Hydrogen peroxide's biocidal action against viruses relies on the oxidation of essential biomolecules that compose the external structures of the virus (i.e. lipid envelope, protein capsid, etc.) [2–4]. Both enveloped and non-enveloped viruses are susceptible to this mechanism, even though non-enveloped viruses are decidedly less susceptible [25]. A recent study indicated that DHP effectively reduced infectious burden of the enveloped coronavirus SARS-CoV-2 on surfaces in a laboratory setting, achieving an estimated 98.7% (1.94 $\log_{10}$) reduction compared to the corresponding control condition after 120 minutes in a simulated room environment [26]. Dry Hydrogen Peroxide was also associated with significant surface reductions in bacteria in two separate studies conducted in active hospital patient rooms [17, 27]. While these studies address DHP's efficacy against bacteria and enveloped viruses on surfaces, there have not yet appeared in the literature peer-reviewed reports detailing the efficacy of DHP against non-enveloped viruses or airborne enveloped viruses. The following sections will detail three previously unpublished laboratory trials that investigated DHP's potential for inactivating airborne viruses or viruses dried on surfaces.

2.4 Efficacy of DHP for inactivating influenza A H1N1

H1N1 is a strain of influenza A (family *Orthomyxoviridae*) that was responsible for a 2009 pandemic declared by the World Health Organization (WHO). Like SARS-CoV-2, H1N1 is an enveloped virus, and it has been known to remain infectious on non-porous surfaces, such as glass and stainless steel, for 24–48 hours

[28, 29]. A DHP device was tested against titers of H1N1, with a starting $TCID_{50}$ of 6.05 log_{10}, in a laboratory biosafety hood to determine if DHP effectively inactivated the virus in comparison to the control condition after 120 minutes exposure (**Tables 1** and **2**).

Aliquots of diluted stock H1N1 were used to inoculate 1″ × 1″ squares on the center of 1″ × 3″ glass slides that had previously been sterilized and autoclaved. The slides were then placed into plastic Petri dishes. Ten slides, in total, were prepared in this way, with duplicates for each timepoint: Time Zero, T = 60 minutes Virus Control, T = 120 minutes Virus Control, T = 60 minutes Virus Test Carrier, T = 120 minutes Virus Test Carrier. Once inoculated with virus, the slides were allowed to dry for 25 minutes at 24°C and 36% relative humidity. The dried carriers were placed in their respective laboratory hoods, one of which was currently being treated with a DHP device that had been operating for 12 hours to precondition the space. The Time Zero samples were immediately collected and eluted with 2 mL of Influenza Infection Medium (EMEM supplemented with 0.125% w/v bovine serum albumin +1 μg/mL TPCK-trypsin + antibiotics). Serial dilutions were then performed to the 10^{-5} dilution and plated in quadruplicate onto MDCK (dog kidney) monolayers. At the designated timepoints, the T = 60 and the T = 120 samples were harvested and enumerated in an identical fashion to the Time Zero samples. The assay trays were then incubated at 35°C on an orbital rotator (60 rotations/minute) for 60 minutes. Once the virus-host cell adsorption had completed, the trays were removed from incubation, and 1.0 mL of the Influenza Infection Medium was pipetted into each well of the assay plate for each of the samples. The MDBK wells were then incubated for 7 days. All titers were determined using the Spearman-Kärber method [30].

After the incubation was complete, the wells were scored for viral cytopathic effect (CPE), and the Tissue Culture Infectivity Dose at the 50% Endpoint Dilution ($TCID_{50}$) was calculated for each pair of samples (**Table 2**). In comparison to the control, the DHP-treated samples yielded a ≥ 2.62 log_{10} reduction in virus titer at 60 minutes and a ≥ 1.87 log_{10} reduction at 120 minutes. The log_{10} reduction in titer observed at 60 minutes corresponds to a percent reduction of ≥99.8%, compared to the control condition (**Table 2**) [31].

Virus	Strain	Cell line	Description	Culture medium
Influenza A (H1N1)[b]	A/PR/8/34	MDCK	Canine Kidney	EMEM +0.125% bovine serum albumin w/v + 1 μg/mL TPCK-trypsin + antibiotics
Feline Calicivirus[c]	ATCC VR-782	CRFK	Feline Kidney	MEM + heat-inactivated fetal bovine serum +100 units/mL penicillin +10 μg/mL gentamicin +2.5 μg/mL amphotericin B
MS2 Bacteriophage[d]	15597-B1	*E. coli* 15597	Gram Negative Bacteria	50% Tryptic Soy Agar

[a]*Abbreviations used: ATCC, American Type Culture Collection; CRFK, Crandel-Reese Feline Kidney; EMEM, Eagle's Minimum Essential Media; MDCK, Madin-Darby Canine Kidney; MEM, Minimum Essential Media.*
[b]*Testing performed at Antimicrobial Test Laboratories, Round Rock, Texas, USA.*
[c]*Testing performed at ATS Labs, Eagan, MN, USA.*
[d]*Testing performed at Microchem Laboratory, Round Rock, TX, USA.*

Table 1.
Summary of viruses and detector cells used in these efficacy studies[a]*.*

	Influenza virus titer ($TCID_{50}$/mL)		
	Time zero	T = 60 min	T = 120 min
Control	6.05	4.80	3.80
DHP-Treated	6.05	≤2.18	≤1.93
Log_{10} Inactivation*		≥2.62	≥1.87
Percent reduction*		≥99.8%	≥98.6%

**Compared to Control.*

Table 2.
Inactivation of influenza virus H1N1 over time by exposure to Dry Hydrogen Peroxide (DHP).

2.5 Efficacy of DHP for inactivating feline calicivirus

Feline calicivirus (FeCV) is a non-enveloped, single-stranded RNA virus (family *Caliciviridae*) that is often used as a surrogate in laboratory testing to simulate human norovirus, a major cause of gastrointestinal hospital-acquired infections (HAIs) [32, 33]. On non-porous surfaces, FeCV has been found to remain viable for 12–72 hours [34]. The efficacy of a prototype DHP device was tested against titers of FeCV, with a starting titer of 6.6 log_{10} $TCID_{50}$/mL, over the course of 24 hours (**Tables 1** and **3**).

Aliquots of FeCV (ATCC VR-782) were inoculated onto glass slides with an accompanying organic soil load of ≤1% fetal bovine serum (FBS) to simulate contamination in a physiological matrix. The original titer of the input virus control was approximately 8.0 log_{10}/mL, but after being allowed to dry on the carriers, the FeCV titer had decreased to an average of 6.6 log_{10}/ml. For both the control and treatment groups, duplicate samples were collected at each timepoint (Time zero, T = 2 hours, T = 6 hours, T = 24 hours). After drying of the virus onto the slides was complete, the carriers were placed in their respective biosafety laboratory hoods, and the DHP device was activated in the hood containing the treatment group of samples. Temperature and humidity levels remained between 21 and 24°C and 36–39%, respectively, throughout the duration of the experiment. The test carriers were retrieved and scraped to resuspend the contents at the designated timepoints. Each sample's contents were transferred to a sterile tube and then serially diluted in the test medium (MEM supplemented with inactivated FBS, 100 units/mL penicillin, gentamicin, and 2.5 μg/mL amphotericin B). Once diluted, a cell-based infectivity assay involving Crandel Reese feline kidney (CRFK) cells was used to determine infectious titer.

The average titer ($TCID_{50}$/mL) for each pair of samples was then calculated (**Table 3**). DHP-treatment resulted in FeCV inactivation (1.5 log_{10} after 2 hours,

	Feline calicivirus titer ($TCID_{50}$/mL)			
	Time zero	T = 2 hr	T = 6 hr	T = 24 hr
Control	6.6	5.8	5.1	3.4
DHP-Treated	6.6	4.3	2.3	≤0.6
Log_{10} Inactivation*		1.5	2.8	≥2.8
Percent reduction*		96.8%	99.8%	≥99.8%

**Compared to Control.*

Table 3.
Inactivation of feline calicivirus over time by exposure to Dry Hydrogen Peroxide (DHP).

and 2.8 log_{10} reduction after 6 hours of exposure time). The 2-hour and 6-hour log_{10} reductions in infectious titer correspond to 96.8% and 99.8% inactivation, respectively, in comparison to the control condition (**Table 3**) [35].

2.6 Efficacy of DHP for inactivating MS2 bacteriophage

MS2 is a single-stranded non-enveloped RNA bacteriophage that often infects *Escherichia coli* (*E. coli*), and has been used as a surrogate for human norovirus and other non-enveloped viruses. MS2 bacteriophage has been shown to survive on non-porous surfaces for 4–10 days, which is aligned with the length of time norovirus can survive under similar conditions [36, 37]. The efficacy of a DHP device against airborne MS2 bacteriophage was investigated over the course of 4 hours (**Tables 1** and **4**).

This trial was conducted in an aerobiology chamber with a volume of ~30 m^3 to simulate the conditions of the DHP device's intended use more accurately. The test inoculum containing a titer (~5.0 log_{10}/mL) of MS2 bacteriophage strain 15597-B1 was split equally and added to two separate nebulizers within the test chamber. These nebulizers were then activated inside the chamber for 60 minutes before the Time Zero sample collection occurred, using an SKC bio-sampler (500 L) equipped with phosphate buffered saline. The sample was then serially diluted and plated in 50% Tryptic Soy Agar (TSA) containing *E. coli* to facilitate the accurate enumeration of the remaining infectious MS2 bacteriophage. Subsequent samples were then collected each hour for the following four hours, with no DHP present, to serve as the no-treatment control. Once the chamber had been adequately decontaminated, the solutions containing the MS2 bacteriophage were again added to the nebulizers. The DHP device was activated after the collection of the Time Zero sample, and subsequent sample collections were performed identically to the control samples. All plated samples were then incubated for 24 hours, and the plaque-forming units (PFU) of MS2 were enumerated. A reduction in log_{10} PFU relative to the untreated control condition is indicative of extent of inactivation.

The Time Zero samples yielded counts of 5.84×10^4 and 5.83×10^4 PFU for the control and DHP-treated groups, respectively. After an hour of exposure to DHP, the count of plaques formed by destroyed *E. coli* decreased by 3.54 log_{10} to 1.70×10^1 PFU, whereas the corresponding untreated control sample decreased by 0.83 log_{10} to 8.61×10^3 PFU. Compared to the untreated control, DHP achieved a 2.71 log_{10} reduction in infectious airborne MS2 bacteriophage titer after 1 hour of exposure, which corresponds to a 99.8% reduction (**Table 4**) [38].

	MS2 bacteriophage titer (*E. coli* PFU/mL)				
	Time zero	**T = 1 hr**	**T = 2 hr**	**T = 3 hr**	**T = 4 hrs**
Control	5.84×10^4	8.61×10^3	2.20×10^3	5.83×10^2	7.59×10^2
DHP-Treated	5.83×10^4	1.70×10^1	$\leq 1.68 \times 10^1$	$\leq 1.58 \times 10^1$	$\leq 1.62 \times 10^1$
Log_{10} Inactivation*		2.70	≥2.12	≥1.57	≥1.67
Percent Reduction*		99.8%	≥99.2%	≥97.3%	≥97.9%

**Compared to control.*

Table 4.
Plaque-forming units (PFU)/mL for E. coli infected with MS2 bacteriophage over time after exposure to Dry Hydrogen Peroxide (DHP).

3. Discussion and conclusions

United States Food and Drug Administration guidance [39] and the literature [40] suggest that small non-enveloped viruses are generally less susceptible to inactivation of germicidal chemicals, such as hydrogen peroxide, than enveloped viruses, vegetative bacteria, and vegetative fungi. The virucidal efficacies displayed in these three surface and air inactivation studies indicate that DHP is capable of reducing surface and air concentrations of both enveloped and non-enveloped viruses. Therefore, it can be reasonably expected that DHP will be capable of similar microbicial efficacy against vegetative bacteria and fungi as well, a hypothesis that is strongly supported by microbial reductions observed in the presence of DHP in healthcare settings [17, 27].

Within healthcare settings, the environmental microbial load is strongly associated with the risk of developing an HAI, and effective reduction of environmental microbial load has been shown to greatly mitigate that risk [41, 42]. It might seem prudent to rely on the most powerful, broad-spectrum disinfectants, such as full-strength VHP, caustics, or chlorine dioxide fogging, which are capable of inactivating pathogens to levels that approach sterile conditions. Those types of disinfectants, unfortunately, can only be applied intermittently. Reliance on intermittent methods of disinfection has repeatedly failed to demonstrate a consistent and effective reduction in environmental bioburden [43]. It is apparent that, for strong disinfectants to achieve their full potential, these must be accompanied by an adjunct method of continuous microbial reduction that can mitigate levels of bioburden during the intervals between the periodic application of the other disinfectants.

In the wake of the SARS-CoV-2 pandemic which caused the COVID-19 disease, there is a unique and universal awareness of the need for effective surface and air hygiene methods in the commercial, educational, and residential sectors. This increased demand for technologies that successfully mitigate environmental pathogen load in sectors outside of healthcare further stresses the need for simple, accessible, and automated adjunct technologies to accompany intermittent microbicidal application protocols and disinfectant usage. The repeated demonstration of the efficacy of DHP against a variety of pathogens in laboratory and field settings, its lack of human toxicity at the H_2O_2 concentrations used, and the material compatibility associated with DHP and its breakdown products (O_2 and H_2O) qualify the technology as a strong contender for meeting this demand.

Author details

Chris Lee[1]* and John R. Henneman[2]

1 EpiClear Consulting, LLC., Columbus, OH, USA

2 Biosecurity Research Institute, Kansas State University, Manhattan, KS, USA

*Address all correspondence to: chris96lee@gmail.com

References

[1] Richardson BW. On peroxide of hydrogen or ozone water as a remedy. Lancet. 1891;i:707-709. doi: 10.1016/S0140-6736(02)19675-9.

[2] McDonnell G, Russell AD. Antiseptics and disinfectants: activity, action and resistance., Clinical Microbiology Reviews. 1999;12:147-179.

[3] Baatout S, De Boever P, Mergeay M. Physiological changes induced in four bacterial strains following oxidative stress. Prikl Biokhim Mikrobiol. 2006;4:418-427.

[4] Peterson HG, Hrudey SE, Cantin IA, et al. Physiological toxicity, cell membrane damage and the release of dissolved organic carbon and geosmin by Aphanizomenon flos-aquae after exposure to water treatment chemicals. Water Research. 1995;29:1515-1523. doi: 10.1016/0043-1354(94)00300-V.

[5] Holmdahl T, Lanbeck P, Wullt M, Walder MH. A head-to-head comparison of hydrogen peroxide vapor and aerosol room decontamination systems. Infection Control & Hospital Epidemiology. 2011;32(9):831-836. doi: 10.1086/661104.

[6] Weber, D. J., Kanamori, H., & Rutala, W. A. 'No touch' technologies for environmental decontamination. Current Opinion in Infectious Diseases. 2016; 29(4): 424-431. doi:10.1097/qco.0000000000000284.

[7] "Occupational health guideline for hydrogen peroxide". US Centers for Disease Control. Retrieved June 2021.

[8] "NIOSH:documentation for immediately dangerous to life or health concentrations". US Centers for Disease Control. Retrieved June 2021.

[9] "Low concentration hydrogen peroxide (LCHP) vapor for bioremediation". Office of Land and Emergency Management. Retrieved June 2021.

[10] "EPA: pesticides - vaporized hydrogen peroxide". US Environmental Protection Agency. Retrieved June 2021.

[11] Falagas, M., Thomaidis, P., Kotsantis, I., Sgouros, K., Samonis, G., & Karageorgopoulos, D. Airborne hydrogen peroxide for disinfection of the hospital environment and infection control: a systematic review. Journal of Hospital Infection. 2011; 78(3): 171-177. doi:10.1016/j.jhin.2010.12.006.

[12] Wijkstrom-Frei C, El-Chemaly S, Ali-Rachedi R, Gerson C, Cobas MA, Forteza R, et al. Lactoperoxidase and human airway host defense. American Journal of Respiratory Cell and Molecular Biology. 2003; 29: 206-212.

[13] Fischer H. Mechanisms and function of DUOX in epithelia of the lung. Antioxidants &Redox Signaling. 2009; 11 (10): 2453-2465.

[14] "Omnia blade HVAC DHP device" and "sphere stand-alone DHP device", Synexis Biodefense, LLC.

[15] Underwriter's Laboratories, Inc. (rep. 1001013827-3432070). Environmental chamber test report for ozone emissions testing. 2020; Marietta, GA.

[16] Underwriter's Laboratories, Inc. (rep. 189477-4180). Environmental claim validation summary. 2020; Marietta, GA.

[17] Marilyn Ramirez, Laura Matheu, Miguel Gomez, Alicia Chang, Jose Ferrolino, Ricardo Mack, Federico Antillon-Klussmann, Mario Melgar. Effectiveness of dry hydrogen peroxide

on reducing environmental microbial bioburden risk in a pediatric oncology intensive care unit. American Journal of Infection Control. 2021; 49(5): 608-613. https://doi.org/10.1016/j.ajic.2020.08.026.

[18] Lee, J. D. Purified hydrogen peroxide gas microbial control methods and devices. 2012 May.

[19] Britigan N, Alshawa A, Nizkorodov SA. Quantification of ozone levels in indoor environments generated by ionization and ozonolysis air purifiers. Journal of Air & Waste Management Association. 2006; 56: 601-610.

[20] ASHRAE Journal. Letter: Changes in IAQ caused by corona discharge air cleaner. 2019.

[21] Daniels SL. Applications of air ionization for control of VOCs and PMx. [Conference presentation] Air and Waste Management Association Conference. 2001; Newport, RI.

[22] Berry D, Mainelis G, Fennell D. Effect of an ionic air cleaner on indoor/outdoor particle ratios in a residential environment. Aerosol Science and Technology. 2007 Apr; 41:3: 315-328. DOI: 10.1080/02786820701199702.

[23] Fink, R. G., & Ellis, W. B. Device, system and method for an advanced oxidation process using photohydroionization. 2005 Aug.

[24] Blake, D. M., Webb, J., Turchi, C., and Magrini, K.; Kinetic and mechanistic overview of TiO2-photocatalyzed oxidationreactions in aqueous solution. Solar Energy Materials. 1991; 24: 584.

[25] Lin, Q., Lim, J. Y., Xue, K., Yew, P. Y., Owh, C., Chee, P. L., & Loh, X. J. Sanitizing agents for virus inactivation and disinfection. 2020; 1(2). https://doi.org/10.1002/viw2.16

[26] Huang, Y.-J. S., Bilyeu, A. N., Hsu, W.-W., Hettenbach, S. M., Willix, J. L., Stewart, S. C., Higgs, S., & Vanlandingham, D. L. Treatment with dry hydrogen peroxide accelerates the decay of severe acute syndrome coronavirus-2 on non-porous hard surfaces. American Journal of Infection Control. 2021. https://doi.org/10.1016/j.ajic.2021.07.006

[27] Sanguinet, J., & Edmiston, C. Evaluation of dry hydrogen peroxide in reducing microbial bioburden in a healthcare facility. American Journal of Infection Control. 2021. https://doi.org/10.1016/j.ajic.2021.03.004.

[28] Oxford, J., Berezin, E. N., Courvalin, P., Dwyer, D. E., Exner, M., Jana, L. A., Kaku, M., Lee, C., Letlape, K., Low, D. E., Madani, T. A., Rubino, J. R., Saini, N., Schoub, B. D., Signorelli, C., Tierno, P. M., & Zhong, X. The survival of influenza A(H1N1)pdm09 virus on 4 household surfaces. American Journal of Infection Control. 2014; 42(4). 423-425. https://doi.org/10.1016/j.ajic.2013.10.016.

[29] Bean, B., Moore, B. M., Sterner, B., Peterson, L. R., Gerding, D. N., & Balfour, H. H. Survival of influenza viruses on environmental surfaces. Journal of Infectious Diseases. 1982; 146(1): 47-51. https://doi.org/10.1093/infdis/146.1.47.

[30] Spearman C. The Method of "Right and wrong cases" (constant stimuli) without Gauss's Formula. British Journal of Psychology. 1908; 2: 227-242.

[31] Antimicrobial Test Laboratories. (rep.). Study report NG3969: custom service time-kill device study to evaluate virucidal efficacy against influenza A (H1N1). 2013. Round Rock, TX.

[32] Gehrke, C., Steinmann, J., & Goroncy-Bermes, P. Inactivation of feline calicivirus, a surrogate of norovirus (formerly Norwalk-like

viruses), by different types of alcohol in vitro and in vivo. Journal of Hospital Infection. 2004; 56(1): 49-55. https://doi.org/10.1016/j.jhin.2003.08.019.

[33] Robilotti, E., Deresinski, S., & Pinsky, B. A. Norovirus. Clinical Microbiology Reviews. 2015; 28(1): 134-164. https://doi.org/10.1128/cmr.00075-14.

[34] Clay, S., Maherchandani, S., Malik, Y. S., & Goyal, S. M. Survival on uncommon fomites of feline calicivirus, a surrogate of noroviruses. American Journal of Infection Control. 2006; 34(1): 41-43. https://doi.org/10.1016/j.ajic.2005.05.013

[35] ATS Labs. (rep.). *A06533:* Virucidal efficacy evaluation of hydrogen peroxide generating unit. 2008. Eagan, MN.

[36] Fisher, E., & Shaffer, R. Survival of bacteriophage MS2 on filtering facepiece respirator coupons. Applied Biosafety. 2010; 15(2): 71-76. https://doi.org/10.1177/153567601001500205.

[37] Leblanc, D., Gagné, M.-J., Poitras, É., & Brassard, J. Persistence of murine norovirus, bovine rotavirus, and hepatitis A virus on stainless steel surfaces, in spring water, and on blueberries. Food Microbiology. 2019; 84: 103257. https://doi.org/10.1016/j.fm.2019.103257.

[38] Microchem Laboratory. (rep.). Study report NG7568: antibacterial activity and aerosol efficacy of Synexis' device. 2016. Round Rock, TX.

[39] Food and Drug Administration. Reprocessing medical devices in health care settings: validation methods and labeling. 2015; 41.

[40] Ijaz, M.K., Nims, R.W., Zhou, S.S. et al. Microbicidal actives with virucidal efficacy against SARS-CoV-2 and other beta- and alpha-coronaviruses and implications for future emerging coronaviruses and other enveloped viruses. Scientific Reports. 2021; 11: 5626.https://doi.org/10.1038/s41598-021-84842-1

[41] Hayden, M. K., Bonten, M. J., Blom, D. W., Lyle, E. A., van de Vijver, D. A., Weinstein, R. A. Reduction in acquisition of vancomycin-resistant enterococcus after enforcement of routine environmental cleaning measures. Clinical Infectious Diseases. 2006; 42(11): 1552-1560. https://doi.org/10.1086/503845.

[42] Denton, M., Wilcox, M. H., Parnell, P., Green, D., Keer, V., Hawkey, P. M., Evans, I., Murphy, P. Role of environmental cleaning in controlling an outbreak of *Acinetobacter baumannii* on a neurosurgical intensive care unit. Journal of Hospital Infection. 2004; 56(2): 106-110. https://doi.org/10.1016/j.jhin.2003.10.017.

[43] Carling PC, Parry MM, Rupp ME, Po JL, Dick B, Von Beheren S; Healthcare Environmental Hygiene Study Group. Improving cleaning of the environment surrounding patients in 36 acute care hospitals. Infection Control & Hospital Epidemiology. 2008 Nov; 29(11):1035-1041. doi: 10.1086/591940.

Chapter 3

Hybrid Hydrogen Peroxide for Viral Disinfection

Meaghan Hislop, Frances Grinstead and John R. Henneman

Abstract

Decontamination is often necessary in facilities with sensitive spaces where pathogen elimination is critical. Historically, high concentration vaporized hydrogen peroxide technologies have been applied in these areas for pathogen disinfection. While effective, these high concentration solutions come with inherent risks to human health and safety. Alternatively, one recent innovation is a hybrid hydrogen peroxide system which combines a 7% hydrogen peroxide solution with a calibrated fogging device that delivers a mixture of vaporous and micro aerosolized particles, significantly lowering the risk of exposure to high-concentration hazardous chemicals. Studies performed with this technology demonstrate high level pathogen decontamination across a variety of tested pathogens and substrates. This chapter will cover a brief history of hydrogen peroxide technologies and their application processes; examine the correlations between viral inactivation, viral disinfection, and biological indicators for validation; demonstrate the necessity of dwell time for optimal efficacy; discuss the effects of viral disinfectant use on laboratory surfaces; and examine various studies, including virologic work performed in Biosafety Level 3 facilities and good laboratory practice (GLP) data performed by EPA-approved laboratories. This chapter will provide readers a deeper understanding of essential components and considerations when implementing hydrogen peroxide systems for viral decontamination.

Keywords: hydrogen peroxide, disinfection, high-level disinfection, decontamination, sterilization, vapor hydrogen peroxide, chlorine dioxide

1. Introduction

Decontamination is a fundamental requirement for research facilities where pathogen elimination is critical, and laboratory facility managers routinely employ various methods of fumigation or fogging disinfection in the never-ending battle against contamination. Historically, technologies such as chlorine dioxide and formaldehyde gas systems have been applied in these areas for pathogen disinfection. Likewise, high concentration vaporized hydrogen peroxide has also been relied on to achieve similar outcomes. A large percentage of these methods follow a familiar pattern of solution injection, dwell (contact time), evacuation, and validation; however, not every system delivers the same functionality or efficacy. Differences in formula and design influence personnel hours, material compatibility, and risk management.

While effective, these high concentration solutions come with inherent risks to health and safety. A recent innovation significantly lowers the risk of exposure to high-concentration chemicals— an HHP™ system which combines a 7% hydrogen peroxide solution with a calibrated fogging device to deliver a mixture of gaseous and micro aerosolized particles. Studies performed with this technology demonstrate high level pathogen disinfection across a variety of tested viruses, bacteria, and substrates. This chapter will provide readers with a deeper understanding of essential components and considerations when implementing systems for viral decontamination. This chapter introduces the latest evolution in hydrogen peroxide disinfection of viral pathogens to address these challenges: an HHP system using patented Pulse™ technology.

1.1 Addressing the need for disinfectants

A dichotomy of virology work is the need for both viral presence within the confines of research and the equally consistent need to establish pathogen-free research spaces. Throughout the world, contagious disease through viral contamination is an ever-present concern, and SARS-CoV-2 has brought the need to decontaminate to the forefront of virtually every industry. Scientific industries performing research, manufacturing pharmaceuticals, or providing healthcare services, all employ protocols for the disinfection of their environments in order for safe, successful, timely work to take place. These industries depend upon disinfection chemicals, and perhaps just as importantly the chemical delivery systems, that ensure the integrity of their work, personnel safety, and efficient transition from one research project or product type to the next.

1.2 Classification of antimicrobial effectiveness

Today, a number of distinct categories are used to classify and understand disinfection methods. Disinfection chemicals are tested with established protocols and classified according to their relative success at eliminating specific pathogens. The *Biosafety in Microbiological and Biomedical Laboratories* (BMBL) 6th edition makes a distinction between the inactivation of pathogens (rendering them non-viable) and the destruction of pathogens and their infectious particles (decontamination) [1]. This distinction is highly relevant to industries where establishing a sterile surface can be a critical determinant of success or failure [2]. The United States Environmental Protection Agency (EPA) classifies disinfectants by their ability to inactivate certain challenging pathogens, such as *Clostridioides difficile* (*C. diff*) and *Bacillus anthracis* (Anthrax), which delineates if the disinfectant is classified a sterilant, decontaminant, or sporicide [3] (**Box 1**). This delineation is based on the Spaulding classification, the microbiological hierarchy model standard, which classifies pathogens based on their environmental hardiness and relative resistance to disinfection [8, 9]. In this hierarchy, small non-enveloped viruses are considered moderately resistant, whereas spores are most resistant to disinfection methods. Beginning in 2016, the EPA developed its Emerging Viral Pathogen category to fast-track products proven against bacterial spores for use against newly appearing viral threats [9–12]. Beyond this classification testing, commercially available spore-based biological indicators can be used with certain solutions as an ongoing measurement and verification of sterilization results [2].

Biosafety in Microbiological and Biomedical Laboratories (BMBL) Definitions [1]	
Decontamination	The use of physical and/or chemical means to remove, inactivate, or destroy microbial pathogens (e.g., bloodborne or aerosolized) on a surface or item to the point where they are no longer capable of transmitting infectious particles and the item or surface is rendered safe to handle: however, this definition has been broadened by infection control specialists to include all pathogens and physical spaces (e.g., patient rooms, laboratories, buildings).
Disinfectant	A substance, or mixture of substances, that destroys or irreversibly inactivates bacteria, fungi, and viruses, but not necessarily bacterial spores or prions, in the inanimate environment.
Disinfection	A process that destroys pathogens and other microorganisms, except prions, by physical or chemical means.
High-Level Disinfection	A lethal process utilizing a sterilant under less than sterilizing conditions (e.g., 10–30 min contact time instead of 6–10 h needed for sterilization). The process kills all forms of microbial life except for large numbers of bacterial spores.
Inactivation	A procedure to render a pathogen non-viable, viral nucleic acid sequences non-infectious, or a toxin non-toxic while retaining characteristic(s) of interest for future use. Methods targeting tropism may be host-specific.
Sterilization	A physical or chemical process that kills or inactivates all microbial life forms including highly resistant bacterial spores.
Sterilant	A substance or mixture of substances that destroys or eliminates all forms of microbial life in the inanimate environment including all forms of vegetative bacteria, bacterial spores, fungi, fungal spores, and viruses.
Validation	Establishment of the performance characteristics of a method and provision of objective evidence that the performance requirements for a specified intended use are fulfilled.
Classification Definitions	
Aerosol	Particulate matter, solid or liquid, larger than a molecule but small enough to remain suspended in the atmosphere [4].
Gas	A substance or matter in a state in which it will expand freely to fill the whole of a container, having no fixed shape (unlike a solid) and no fixed volume (unlike a liquid) [5].
Hybrid H_2O_2	A mixture of gaseous and micro aerosolized substance which remain suspended in the air to fill the whole container [6]
Vapor	A substance diffused or suspended in the air, especially one normally liquid or solid [7].

Box 1.
Definitions. *Definitions relating to achieving and evaluating levels of antimicrobial effectiveness on environmental surfaces [1]. Definitions of substance phase or classification [4–7]. Depending on device design, the chemical being dispersed throughout the treatment space may be delivered in a variety of forms, phases, or states of matter. These definitions are provided for the sake of our understanding the differences in technologies and delivery methods described within this chapter.*

1.3 The evolution of disinfection systems

One growing understanding is that the application method of a disinfectant plays a critical role in the success of the disinfection results. While some of the most common spray and wipe surface disinfectants have been in use for decades, there are challenges to their application which can result in inconsistent or ineffective results. Adequate distribution and required contact time are difficult to achieve on a consistent basis by hand application methods, especially in large spaces with high ceilings and complex surface profiles. These accessibility issues and failures may result in inconsistent and incomplete elimination of surface contamination [13]. To address inherent inconsistencies in manual disinfection and to provide alternative methods of delivery, various technologies have been applied. Those technologies include fumigation with formaldehyde, chlorine dioxide gas, fogging of hydrogen peroxide as vapor, silver hydrogen peroxide systems, and hybrid hydrogen peroxide systems. Their gaseous and vaporous form allows access to, and contact with, surfaces that spray and wipe methods alone often cannot access. Automated systems have taken these chemicals with known disinfectant action and paired them with dispersion devices, aiming to deliver an appropriate contact time and maximize surface exposure. These systems automate much of the disinfection process, helping to remove human error and mitigate safety concerns from contact with potentially caustic chemicals. In particular, H_2O_2-based systems have become a front-runner among automated high-level disinfection technologies due to H_2O_2's effectiveness, material compatibilities, lack of chemical residues, and increased safety over other technologies such as formaldehyde or chlorine dioxide gas [14–18]. When applied in multiple life science environments, H_2O_2 fogging is well documented to have efficacy against numerous viral pathogens and has seen a rise in use in environments where thorough efficacy and decontamination of a room and its contents are needed [19–22].

1.4 Mechanism of action of hydrogen peroxide

Anyone who has skinned their knee and poured hydrogen peroxide on the wound to stave off infection is familiar with the use of H_2O_2 as an antiseptic and anti-bacterial agent. Indeed, hydrogen peroxide is produced naturally in the body, acting as a beacon triggering the accumulation of white blood cells of the immune response [23]. Hydrogen Peroxide was first discovered in 1818 by Louis Jacque Theénard, who described it as 'eau oxygénéé or water oxygen for its composition containing one more oxygen atom than water [24]. This single oxygen–oxygen or peroxide bond is naturally unstable and prone to decomposition with or without the presence of a catalyst [25]. During decomposition, the active oxygen atom cleaves off, releasing energy and resulting in water and oxygen molecules [26]. The oxidizing activity, resulting from the presence of the extra oxygen atom, is what makes hydrogen peroxide an effective disinfectant. It is the reactive formulation of hydrogen peroxide which causes destruction of pathogens by breaking apart structures, interrupting key functions, causing damage to DNA, and eliminating infectious particles.

2. Hybrid hydrogen peroxide via pulse technology

One of the biggest challenges to any disinfectant application is ensuring a thorough and consistent disinfectant exposure to contaminated surfaces for an effective contact time. To achieve success, fogging technologies must perform a complicated dance between the amount of chemical injected, temperature, humidity, dew point, and method, all of which can affect efficacy from one application to the next. To answer this need, CURIS System designed and patented the concept of replenishing any naturally decomposing solution and called it Pulse technology, simplifying the complicated balance of a successful disinfection. Combining a 7% hydrogen peroxide solution with a calibrated fogging device, this HHP system delivers hybrid hydrogen peroxide, a mixture of gaseous and micro aerosol particles. While effective in a liquid solution, fogging with hydrogen peroxide in this hybrid form increases the availability of each H_2O_2 molecule, maximizing oxidation opportunities and leading to the destruction of pathogens on surfaces. Beyond just inactivating pathogens, this oxidation causes a physical destructive action of pathogen components, which further delineates this substance as a decontaminant as defined by the BMBL.

A fundamental distinction of this system is its ability to disperse a lower concentration of 7% hydrogen peroxide at calibrated intervals, maximizing contact time while using less H_2O_2 to achieve microbicidal efficacy. The HHP device operates by delivering the HHP mixture in a two-part process. First, it fills an enclosure with disinfecting fog to an optimal level for killing pathogens. Second, it maintains the fog at the optimal level without oversaturation by periodically injecting more solution into the space being treated, and thereby prolonging the active contact time of the H_2O_2 (**Figure 1**). This not only helps to keep surfaces dry, it also reduces sensitivity to variations in temperature and other factors. One might consider this similar to cruise control in a vehicle—the initial phase continuously revs the engine to get the vehicle up to speed, while the second phase uses the engine just enough to keep it at the cruising speed without exceeding the limit. In the case of disinfection, it means keeping the fog concentration at the optimum "kill" level to achieve efficacy in a relatively short time, yet without exceeding this optimum level to the point where the fog condenses on surfaces in the treatment area.

2.1 Chemical concentrations and safety implications

With a concentration of 7% H_2O_2, the solution, known as CURoxide™, is below the 8% hazard threshold [27, 28]. Being below the threshold means special shipping considerations are not required. Moreover, this enables safer handling for personnel than the 35–59% H_2O_2 solutions traditionally employed for fogging applications [18, 29–31]. Likewise, the 7% solution is safer for laboratory materials than the 28.1–52% concentration of corrosive industrial strength grade hydrogen peroxide [27, 32]. This material safety (compatibility) is perhaps most evident when

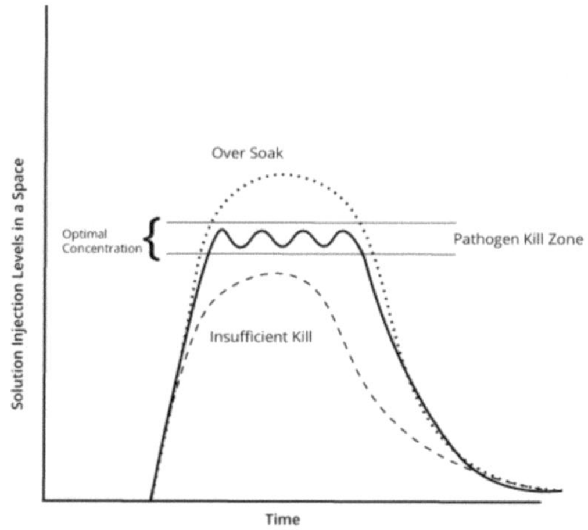

Figure 1.
Pulse HHP Cycle. *Hydrogen peroxide released as a vapor or aerosol begins a natural decomposition into water and oxygen within 10 minutes. Most fogging delivery methods require longer contact time. Pulse technology periodically replenishes active hydrogen peroxide during the decontamination cycle, prolonging the effective contact time, and promoting an optimal pathogen kill zone.*

considering how the hydrogen peroxide concentration of a solution will evolve when the solution transitions through states of matter. Hydrogen peroxide is more resistant to leaving the liquid state and more likely to return to it than the water in the solution. When transitioning from vapor back into liquid, this can result in surface condensation at more than double the initial liquid concentration (**Figure 2**). At 7% H_2O_2, the HHP solution remains below the 45% known level of material incompatibility [33].

The levels of particle concentration used in typical high-level disinfection are of particular concern to facility managers. These concerns may be lessened by employing lower particle-producing products. Technologies utilizing formaldehyde, chlorine dioxide, and high concentration H_2O_2 operate at concentrations as high as 1,400 parts per million (ppm) [34–36]. By contrast, the HHP 7% solution has a lower operating concentration of approximately 138 ppm [37]. Traditional vaporized approaches require a concentration that is up to 10× higher than the lower 7% H_2O_2 concentration enables, which accordingly may result in a greater risk to personnel from leakage with typical high concentration systems [38]. This is particularly important because, according to the National Library of Medicine, "Inhalation of vapors from concentrated (greater than 10%) solutions may result in severe pulmonary irritation" [39]. This may be why there is a substantial safety concern among facility managers when it comes to typical fogging approaches, as these approaches utilize caustic chemicals at very high concentrations which are known to penetrate through gaps as small as a keyhole [38, 40].

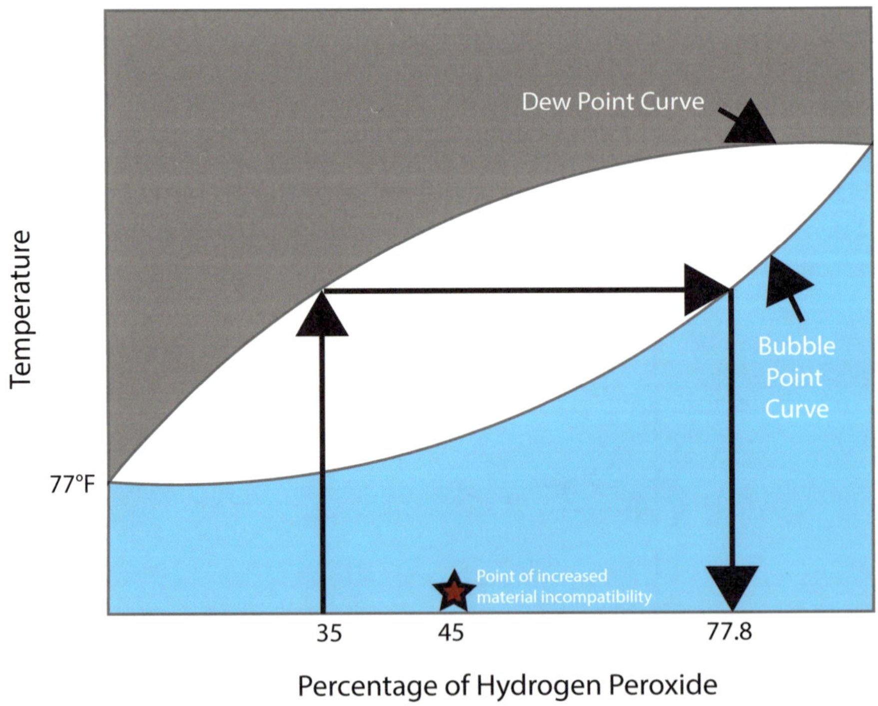

Figure 2.
Fluctuations in H_2O_2 Concentration. *Adapted from Hultman et al. [33] the concentration of hydrogen peroxide changes throughout different states of matter. When vapor condenses onto a surface the peroxide is more likely to enter the liquid state than the water vapor. This results in surface concentrations significantly higher than the original solution concentration. Concentrations exceeding 45% H_2O_2 are higher than the recommended maximum concentration for suitable interaction with other materials. In this manner a 35% solution that has been vaporized and condensed out on surfaces can reach concentrations of 77.8% H_2O_2 [33].*

2.2 HHP device description

Roughly the size of a small suitcase, the 36-pound (16 kg) HHP system fogs enclosures from an adjustable stainless-steel nozzle at the top of the unit. It can be wheeled or carried throughout a facility to disinfect a wide variety of spaces, large or small, and its Rotomold design provides durability for long-term use and sturdiness during transport. A push-button design allows users to input area dimensions through the device's manual digital interface, or users may operate the device remotely via a tablet for touchless disinfection from outside the treatment space. The system self-calculates the cubic footage of the space to be fogged to determine the amount of disinfectant needed, and an indicator light shows users when the appropriate amount of solution has been added to the reservoir. An electronically sequenced A/C electrical outlet provides optional connection for any desired additional equipment.

2.3 Smart technology

In a world where everything is documented to defend, reinforce, train, and track information, technologies with the ability to employ these methods are invaluable to present and future decontamination applications. The HHP system incorporates patented smart technology, allowing operation not only from a device interface but also remotely through its control app for phones and tablets (**Figure 3**). For larger spaces, multiple devices may simultaneously work together via wireless communication to combine their capacities to fill the larger volume without the added complications of cables. Whether used alone or in a network, the fogging device(s) self-calculates the dosage required for a space once dimensions are provided. For each disinfection cycle, a job report is wirelessly generated and saved into a secure data system, providing the facility with trackable records in support of risk management protocols. On-demand training, reference materials, and technical support are also available through this secure data storage system, which includes security codes, usernames, and password protection against unauthorized operation and modifications. These smart technology components give laboratory personnel the

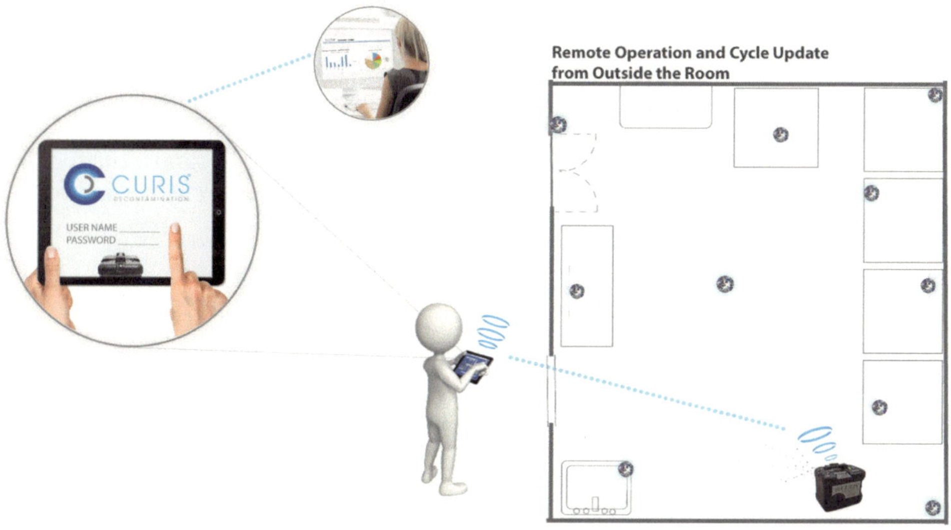

Figure 3.
Hybrid Hydrogen Peroxide (HHP) Smart Technology. *Wireless remote operation via tablet, with secure data management. The HHP device is operated from outside the enclosure. Once the treatment cycle is complete, the data are uploaded and recorded to a secure database for customer analytics and job reports.*

ability to remotely operate and monitor the system, lessening concerns affiliated with exposure to high concentrations of H_2O_2.

2.4 Versatility

2.4.1 Large enclosure decontamination

The HHP device offers the ability to decontaminate enclosed spaces as large as 14,000 ft^3 (396 m^3) by itself or wirelessly pair up to 25 devices together to treat spaces as large as 350,000 ft^3 (9,911 m^3) at once. Although the EPA approvals are for 3,682 ft^3 (103 m^3) due to the size limitation of the testing laboratory, efficacy of bacterial spores are documented in much larger spaces [41]. The small, compact design also reaches tall ceilings efficaciously, as noted in studies where 6-$\log_{10}$ reductions of *Geobacillus stearothermophilus* challenged indicators were proven at 21 ft. However, all treated spaces are to be validated with 6-$\log_{10}$ biological indicators for optimal application.

2.4.2 Attachments

Since many life science facilities are made up of diversely sized spaces and needs, the next generation of Pulse technology device was developed. Retaining the core fogging unit's design, the new attachment model offers the ability to fog, hand spray, or port in, all from the same unit. This fogging model can disinfect large open spaces with a hand sprayer (with proper personal protective equipment). The device can also port into enclosed spaces, such as labs or mobile equipment, with extension nozzles, or it can connect to various enclosures found within laboratories.

2.4.3 Scalable decontamination

To enable decontamination of small enclosures, the HHP system pairs with a mobile cart designed to attach to biological safety cabinets, isolators, incubators, filters, and filter housings (**Figure 4a**) [42]. This modular pairing delivers low concentration H_2O_2 solution to the closed system environment, extracts vapor once decontamination has been achieved, and conditions the space to return it to its normal operating environment. No disassembly of lab equipment is required. The system achieves decontamination of the entire chamber, including filters, and contents. The rolling cart weighs approximately 50 pounds (22 kg) and includes a pullout tray to house the HHP fogging device. For scalable applications, the fogging device can fog a whole laboratory or be coupled to the mobile cart as needed for smaller enclosures.

2.4.4 Facility integration

The HHP system also enables integration with a laboratory or stand-alone chamber. This modular design allows for custom installation into facilities—including integrated nozzles and touchscreen operation—to provide decontamination to these essential spaces (**Figure 4b**). For facilities requiring unified operation of environmental or electronic controls, the HHP system works in tandem with smart integration technology to provide remote operation, automation, and mounted disinfection for one or more enclosed spaces at a time. Decontamination chamber or washer integration includes cycles of less than 120 minutes, including aeration. This chamber integration enables users to operate the entire chamber from one common point, the display screen. It is suitable for coupling with chambers from a variety of manufacturers.

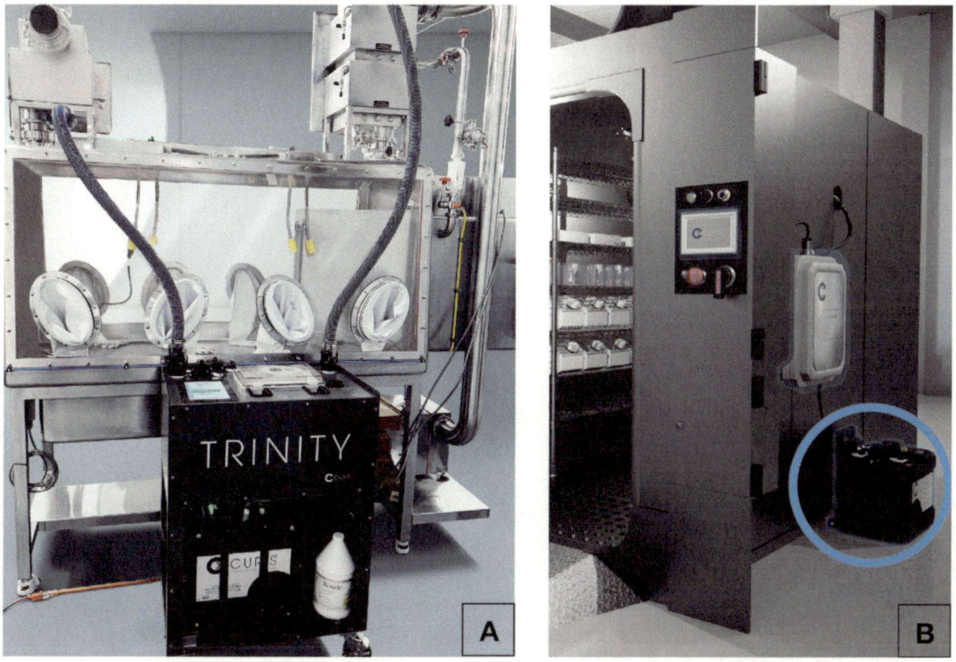

Figure 4.
Scalability and Integration. *A. Modular cart coupled with hybrid hydrogen peroxide (HHP) device, shown here decontaminating a glove box. B. HHP system integration for decontamination of a laboratory or chamber and its contents.*

2.4.5 HHP applications

During the 2020–2021 COVID-19 pandemic, the HHP system was approved by the EPA for use against SARS-CoV-2 through the Emerging Viral Pathogen designation due to its sporicidal efficacy [37]. As a result, the HHP system was used in many different environments as a tool for mitigating risk to personnel, research, and equipment. Healthcare facilities faced with shortages of personal protective equipment (PPE) employed the system to decontaminate and safely reuse PPE until the supply could be reestablished. Life science facilities incorporated the HHP system for decontaminating manufacturing spaces where vaccine work was taking place. The HHP system was also instrumental in multiple military applications, significantly aided by the portable design and accessible use. Some prior and ongoing uses include disinfection of manufacturing facilities with a need for sterilization, sterile processing facilities, drug manufacturing facilities, vivariums, laboratory contents, laboratories with interstitial spaces, laboratory filter housings, compounding pharmacies, surgical suites, healthcare patient rooms, ambulances, equipment for service providers, biological safety cabinets, isolator filters, and gnotobiotics.

3. HHP testing efficacy data

3.1 Introduction

Studies performed with Pulse technology demonstrate high-level pathogen disinfection across a variety of tested viruses, bacteria, and bacterial spores. The data presented here include a mixture of peer-reviewed studies, Good Laboratory Practice (GLP)-regulated testing, and real-world applications where disinfection can be further complicated by condition-dependent factors such as biofilms, soil loads, and surface type (porous/non-porous), all of which can protect and harbor infectious pathogens [13, 43]. Across the body of this work, the target of high-level disinfection is not only to reduce the present contamination, but to reduce it sufficiently to prevent an infectious dose or the potential for colony regrowth. The work presented here demonstrates the HHP system's ability to decontaminate, destroying microbial pathogens. This complete decontamination is critical as any surviving pathogens have the potential to interfere with or invalidate research, contaminate sterile products, and cause health hazards.

3.2 Validating the HHP process

When targeting pathogens invisible to the eye, there must be some way to measure the efficacy of disinfection. Employing validation tools gives the ability to verify a disinfection process using living organisms and giving results rooted in science. Though several types of chemical and pH indicators exist, indicators of *Geobacillus stearothermophilus* bacterial spores (1×10^6 organisms) are used as the international standard for validation of sterilization by hydrogen peroxide [44, 45]. These 6-$\log_{10}$ indicators consist of a verified population of approximately 1 million bacterial spores. The evolutionary hardiness of bacterial spores has led to them being used as a standard of measurement for sterilization [2]. Inactivation of these difficult-to-penetrate spores also represents confirmation of efficacy in disinfecting lower-level pathogens, such as non-enveloped viruses, gram-negative and gram-positive bacteria, molds, yeasts, and enveloped viruses (**Figure 5**) [8, 9, 45]. Likewise, proving inactivation of these robust organisms predicts successful disinfection of more susceptible pathogens [11, 12].

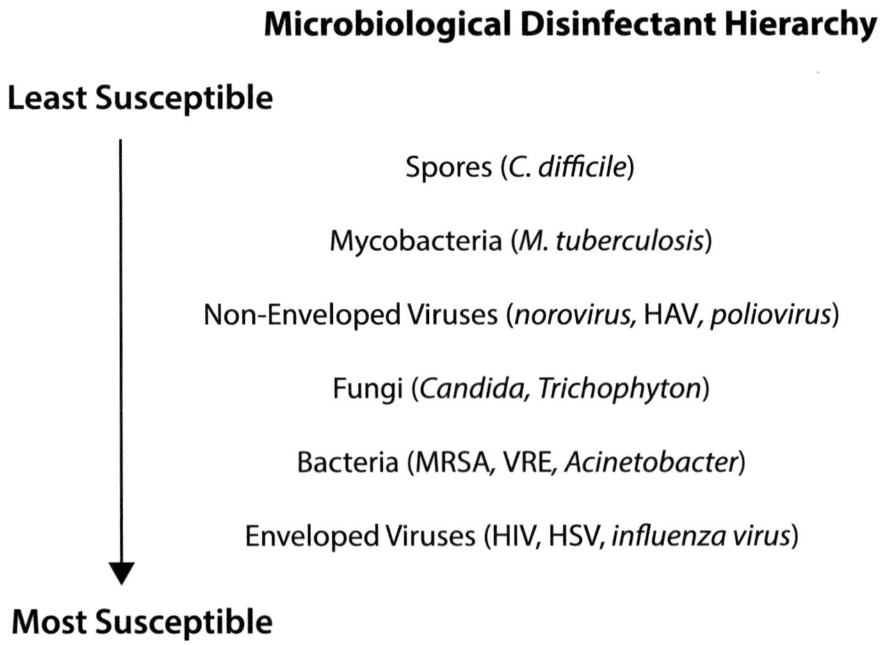

Figure 5.
Microbiological Disinfection Hierarchy. *Described in* chemical disinfection of medical and surgical materials, *EH Spaulding ranked the microbiological hierarchy of disinfectants, listing organisms from least susceptible to most susceptible, according to their vulnerability to disinfectants [8, 9, 45].*

Recognizing a disinfectant's ability to kill less susceptible pathogens as an indicator of broader effectiveness, the EPA offers a variety of specific designations a chemical or system can claim. In 2018, the HHP system was approved for sporicidal classification by the EPA for a 6-log_{10} reduction of *Clostridioides difficile* (*C. diff*) in a tripartite soil load [46]. The EPA's Emerging Viral Pathogens claim was additionally approved for the HHP system on the basis of this sporicidal data [37]. Granting of this classification may further support the validity that efficacy against bacterial spores will likely conclude efficacy against enveloped and non-enveloped viruses. Targeting a 6-log_{10} or greater reduction of bacterial spores for validation is a key component of achieving a successful high-level disinfection [47]. Achieving this 6-log_{10} sporicidal kill will enable confidence against more susceptible organisms, such as enveloped or non-enveloped viruses [9] which may exist in a soil load or biofilm, making them more difficult to inactivate [13, 43].

3.3 Viral efficacy data: norovirus

Norovirus, a single stranded non-enveloped virus of the Caliciviridae family, is a leading cause of acute gastroenteritis in humans. The most common genogroup GII is responsible for 95% of infections, which can have severe and even fatal outcomes in at-risk populations such as young children or the elderly. Norovirus, once present, can become a pervasive problem due to the environmental stability of the virus, low infectious dose, resistance to alcohol and chlorine-based disinfectants, and the potential for prolonged asymptomatic shedding of infected individuals. Norovirus is also used as a target organism for testing, as it is considered to be a non-enveloped virus with relatively low susceptibility to disinfectants [48].

In 2018, a 1,600-bed assisted living facility had a norovirus outbreak affecting 1/4 of the residents within a 2-week period with an average of 40 new cases a day, despite protective measures such as the quarantine of afflicted individuals. A bio-decontamination company employing HHP technology was brought into the facility for outbreak response and control. HHP fogging was implemented as part of a 5-point process including continued quarantine and enhanced staff education. After a four-day implementation period, no new cases were reported, effectively ending the outbreak [49].

The HHP system was also tested under GLP conditions for efficacy against the norovirus testing surrogate feline calicivirus [20]. In this testing, 21 inoculated glass agar carrier plates were placed throughout the test room, ranging from floor level to 12 feet (3.6 m) in height, and exposed to the HHP fogging protocols. There was no recovered virus from the challenged plates for an overall reduction of 7.6 log_{10} (**Table 1**). Interestingly, efficacious results were also noted in GLP compliant testing when a carrier plate lid was accidentally left on during the HHP fogging cycle. This protocol deviation allowed for the observation that, even under these challenging conditions, the HHP fog migrated underneath the lid and achieved inactivation of viral particles [20].

The combination of these two studies demonstrates that the HHP system effectively disinfects complex spaces contaminated with norovirus or its surrogates in both laboratory and real-world conditions. Though the assisted living facility case study did not measure a numerical reduction of viral burden, the effective outbreak control of 100% reduction in new cases leads to the conclusion that norovirus was reduced to levels less than the infectious dose.

3.4 Viral efficacy data: within porous materials

In the spring/summer of 2020, the COVID-19 pandemic triggered a scarcity, and subsequent shortage of personal protective equipment (PPE) used by hospitals and

HHP Efficacy				
Pathogen [reference]	**Characteristics**	**Strain/ Source**	**Carrier Type**	**Results**
Bacillus subtilis [50]	Gram-positive, rod-shaped, endospore formation	19615	Dacron suture loop Porcelain Penicylinders (50% Tyvek/Tyvek)	75 of 77 carriers negative 5.2 $\log_{10}$ reduction (Penicylinder) 6.2 $\log_{10}$ reduction (suture)
Clostridium sporogenes [50]	Gram-positive, rod-shaped, endospore formation	3584	Dacron suture loop Porcelain Penicylinders (50% Tyvek/Tyvek)	73 of 74 carriers negative 6.1 $\log_{10}$ reduction (Penicylinder) 6.3 $\log_{10}$ reduction (suture)
Geobacillus stearothermophilus [41]	Gram-positive, rod-shaped, endospore formation	ATCC 7953	Tyvek/Tyvek stainless steel coupon	206 carriers negative 6.2 $\log_{10}$ reduction
Clostridioides difficile [46]	Gram-positive, rod-shaped, endospore formation	ATCC 43598	Stainless Steel Disk	90 carriers negative 6.6 $\log_{10}$ reduction
***Pseudomonas* phi6 (phi6)** [19]	Enveloped, icosahedral	phi 6	Porous N95 Mask	36 of 37 $\geq$ 6.0 $\log_{10}$ reduction*
Norovirus [49]	Non-enveloped, icosahedral	Unknown	Wild type	100% reduction of cases
Feline calicivirus (U.S. EPA-approved norovirus surrogate) [20]	Non-enveloped, icosahedral	Strain F-9, ATCC VF-782	Glass Petri Dish	40 of 40 plates $\geq$7.58 $\log_{10}$ reduction
Herpes simplex virus 1 (HSV-1) [19]	Enveloped, icosahedral	Strain F	Porous N95 Mask	64 of 65 $\geq$ 5 $\log_{10}$ reduction*
Coxsackievirus B3 (CVB3) [19]	Non-enveloped (naked), icosahedral	Strain B3	Porous N95 Mask	6o of 63 $\geq$ 4.3 $\log_{10}$ reduction*
SARS-CoV-2 [19]	Enveloped, no icosahedral capsid	Isolate USA-WA1/ 2020	Porous N95 Mask	48 of 48 reduced below LOD

Table 1.
***Efficacy**. Summary table of data presented within this chapter demonstrating efficacy of the HHP system against a range of pathogens and substrates. Sporicidal results show inactivated (negative) carriers by log reduction, viral results show either log reduction or limit of detection (LOD) where applicable. * indicates where $\log_{10}$ reduction is the starting log titer and the LOD = log titer.*

other healthcare facilities. In an attempt to find ways to mitigate this emergency, researchers at Pennsylvania State University (Penn State) employed HHP to disinfect expired N95 respirators to assess the applicability of the HHP system for this use. Respirators were tested both for any physical degradation effects of the treatment on the respirator material and for efficacy of disinfection of respirator components via inoculation with three viral pathogens and one bacteriophage. Viral work performed at the Eva J Pell Biosafety Level 3 laboratory at Penn State used viruses of different characteristics, as well as a bacteriophage, to represent the range of physical characteristics of pathogens to which healthcare workers may be exposed (**Table 1**) [19]. Three viruses: herpes simplex virus (HSV-1; enveloped virus; family Herpesviridae), coxsackievirus (CVB3; non-enveloped virus; family Picornaviridae), and SARS-CoV-2 (isolate USA-WA1/2020; enveloped virus; family Coronaviridae), as well as pseudomonas bacteriophage (phi6; enveloped), were chosen for testing (**Figure 6**). The inside, outside, and strap materials of the respirators were used as inoculation sites. While the majority of these surfaces are made up of porous materials, at least one type of respirator had an outer layer of hydrophobic material which caused the inoculation droplet to dry into a 'coffee ring' pattern on the respirator. This testing of porous materials is significant because it presents a more difficult challenge to disinfection than non-porous surfaces, since the materials which absorb the pathogen may also provide a degree of protection, at least temporarily [51]. Disinfectant efficacy testing is commonly done on non-porous surfaces, which does not reflect the difficulty and variables that porous surfaces present.

Testing performed at Penn State also included the use of biological indicators as validation of the protocol for a successful HHP cycle. For each HHP cycle, 6 to 12 biological indicators (*Geobacillus stearothermophilus* ATCC® 7953) with a mean spore count 2.4×10^5 on stainless steel carriers encased in Tyvek®/Glassine pouches were placed throughout the room. In the total of 14 disinfection cycles, only 2 of 138 indicators returned positive for spore growth. These included preliminary cycles, which were intended to establish optimal cycle parameters [19].

3.5 Viral efficacy indicated through bacterial spore validation

The EPA and the Centers for Disease Control and Prevention (CDC) recognize that certain microorganisms can be ranked with respect to their tolerance to chemical disinfectants [7]. As a result, efficacy against less susceptible bacterial spores can be extrapolated to indicate efficacy against more susceptible microorganisms, including enveloped and non-enveloped viruses [8, 9, 52].

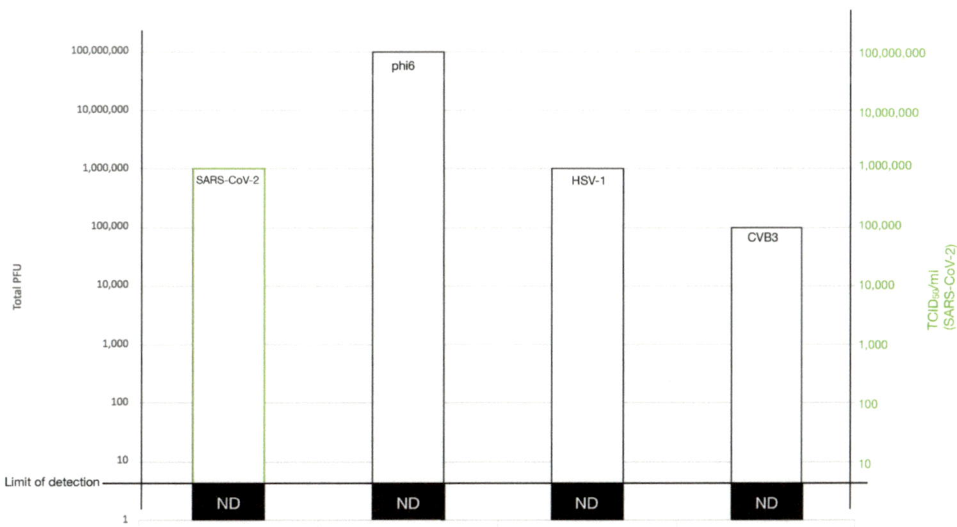

■ Post-Fogging Detection	0	0	0	0
□ Pre-Fogging Count	1,000,000	100,000,000	1,000,000	100,000
Reduction	≥1,000,000 $TCID_{50}$/ml	6 $\log_{10}$	5 $\log_{10}$	4.3 $\log_{10}$
	Cycle # Post 2	Cycle # Post 1	Cycle # Post 1	Cycle # Post 1

Figure 6.
Viral Reductions Post Hybrid Hydrogen Peroxide (HHP) Fogging. *Data table demonstrating the efficacy of HHP fogging for reducing tested viruses and bacteriophage to below the limit of detection–not detected (ND)–measured as either plaque-forming units (PFU) or median tissue culture infectious dose ($TCID_{50}$) [19].*

3.5.1 Bacterial spore efficacy data: necropsy, laboratories, and interstitial spaces

To assess efficacy within various Biosafety Level 3 Agricultural (BSL-3Ag) environments, Kansas State University challenged the HHP system within their Biosecurity Research Institute, a BSL-3Ag facility. Testing was performed in three laboratories representing a range of sizes: 2,281 ft^3 (65 m^3), 4,668 ft^3 (132 m^3), and 44,212 ft^3 (1,252 m^3). Each of the two smaller laboratories were tested over a series of three disinfection cycles with biological indicators of *Geobacillus stearothermophilus* (6.2 $\log_{10}$ spores) encased in Tyvek/Tyvek and placed throughout the laboratories, in laboratory equipment such as biological safety cabinets, and in the overhead interstitial space (drop ceiling). Testing in these laboratories resulted in a greater than 6-$\log_{10}$ reduction of all 252 challenged indicators, including those placed in the difficult to access interstitial space.

Within the largest space tested, the 44,212 ft^3 (1,252 m^3) necropsy laboratory, four HHP devices were used for the disinfection cycle. The smart technology of the HHP system automated the connection of multiple Pulse fogging devices for a synchronized, custom-calibrated, HHP cycle. A total of 206 biological indicators were tested over two HHP cycles in locations throughout the laboratory, including at the 21-ft (6.4 m) ceiling height, soft-sided anteroom, walk-in cooler, and change rooms. All 206 challenged indicators were negative for spore growth, demonstrating a greater than 6-$\log_{10}$ reduction of *G. stearothermophilus*. This BSL-3Ag testing provides real-life results within the targeted environment for the HHP system. The smart controls and automation allowed this testing to be performed in house by the laboratory personnel [41].

3.5.2 Bacterial spore efficacy data: sterilization study on porous surfaces

The BMBL (6th edition) defines sterilization as; "a physical or chemical process that kills or inactivates all microbial life forms including highly resistant bacterial spores." The importance of sterilization is well understood in life science, pharmaceutical, and healthcare industries. Through the process of sterilization, researchers and physicians alike establish the basis for reliable and safe protocols and procedures. Standards for fogging sterilization testing are developed by the Association of Official Analytical Chemists (AOAC International), a globally recognized, third party not-for-profit, that provides education and facilitates the development of test methods and standards.

The HHP system was challenged with the Fogging Devices Sterilant Test (OCSPP 810.2100) for efficacy against *B. subtilis* (strain 19615) spores, an opportunistic pathogen, which is tolerant of ultraviolet light and high temperatures, and *Clostridium sporogenes* (strain 3584) spores, a strain of *Clostridium botulinum*. These two spores are designated for this test due to their enhanced survivability compared to other spore types. Two carrier formations were used for both spore types, porcelain Penicylinders and Dacron™ suture loops. Each carrier type was saturated with the substrate, distributing spores throughout these materials. Half of each type of carrier was placed inside Tyvek/Tyvek pouches, with the remaining carriers placed in glass petri dishes. Carriers with these bacterial spores were placed throughout the 9′11″ × 14′6″ × 12′9″ (1,833 ft^3 / 51 m^3) testing room. A total of 151 carriers were tested, with only three carriers being found positive for spore growth, all on porcelain Penicyliner carriers enclosed in Tyvek/Tyvek pouches (1 *B. subtilis*, 2 *C. sporogenes*) [50]. This testing method is designed to challenge a fogging system's penetration and subsequent disinfection of spores within these porous carriers. These results demonstrated the HHP system's ability to penetrate through two forms of porous surfaces to inactivate the resistant spores.

3.5.3 Bacterial spore efficacy data: sporicidal study in a tripartite soil load

Clostridioides difficile is a bacterium responsible for causing almost half a million infections in the United States alone each year, with fatal outcomes for 1 in 11 people over the age of 65 within one month of infection [53]. *Clostridioides difficile (C. diff)* is considered one of the most epidemiologically important pathogens, as its environmental persistence, antibiotic resistance, and low infectious dose have led to this bacterium plaguing hospitals and long-term care facilities alike [54]. Precisely due to the hardiness of this bacterium in spore form, *C. diff* has become a standard against which to measure disinfectant efficacy and forms the basis of the EPA's Emerging Viral Pathogen efficacy and approval [12]. With the understanding that pathogens in the environment do not exist in a vacuum, but rather are more likely to be found within a soil load consisting of physiological fluids such as blood, purulent material, or feces, the EPA updated testing requirements for sporicidal classification to challenge not only against hardy *C. diff* spores, but to test such spores within three protective materials (tripartite load; bovine serum albumin, yeast extract, mucin). In 2018, the HHP system was awarded sporicidal classification in the EPA's most stringent *C. diff* test; elimination of *C. diff* spores in a tripartite soil load. A total of 63 carrier plates over three testing lots were exposed to the HHP cycle, resulting in the inactivation of all 63 carriers and an average $\log_{10}$ reduction of 6.6 for this difficult to kill bacterial spore. This testing confirmed the HHP system's ability for high-level disinfection with sporicidal classification [46].

4. Comparison to existing technologies

4.1 Fumigated formaldehyde devices

Formaldehyde is a naturally occurring compound consisting of hydrogen, oxygen, and carbon which is used as a disinfectant in both its liquid and gaseous states [55]. Used as a laboratory fumigant since the late 19th century, formaldehyde has remained in use due to its efficacy and low cost [56, 57]. For use as a disinfectant, formalin, the aqueous form of formaldehyde, is heated into a vapor producing formaldehyde gas [58]. When encountering microbes, this gas causes a cross-linking of molecules leading to protein clumping and loss of structure [59]. While an effective sterilant, formaldehyde must be handled with extreme care as exposure can cause asthma-like respiratory problems, cancer, or even be fatal to humans [55]. In gaseous form, formaldehyde is used at 8,000–10,000 ppm concentration and leaves behind a residue which must be removed through manual cleaning [56, 60]. Due to the potential health hazards and the required labor-intensive clean-up of residue, formaldehyde use is declining in favor of less hazardous and faster solutions. Indeed, the European Union lists formaldehyde as a substance of very high concern and has issued regulation calling for the progressive substitution when suitable alternatives have been identified [61]. While generally compatible with laboratory materials, formaldehyde can be absorbed into porous materials such as HEPA filters, off-gassing slowly and extending the time needed for safe re-entry [56, 62]. Formaldehyde production equipment ranges from as small as an electric fry pan requiring timers or externally controlled circuits to larger automated devices roughly the size of a household refrigerator and weighing approximately 396 pounds (180 kg) [63].

4.2 Chlorine dioxide devices

Chlorine dioxide (ClO_2) is a synthetic, green-colored gas that gives off a bleach-like odor. Despite the familiar scent, chlorine dioxide gas is toxic and must be carefully contained when employed as a fumigant [64]. Consisting of unstable chlorine (Cl_2) and oxygen molecules (O_2), ClO_2 disassociates when heated into chloride (Cl-), chlorite (ClO-) and chlorate ions (ClO_3-). Some formulations can leave residues of sodium chlorite or inert salts, such as sodium chloride, on surfaces [65]. The disinfection cycle for ClO_2 commonly consists of five steps: pre-conditioning, conditioning, charge (gas injection), exposure (contact time), and aeration [66]. The cycle is humidity-dependent, requiring a dosage increase of approximately 500 ppm for each 10% change in humidity, leading to an operating concentration range of 600–1550 ppm [66]. Similar to formaldehyde, ClO_2 can be absorbed into porous surfaces and thus take longer to aerate than non-porous materials [65]. One consideration for system use is material compatibility with laboratory equipment. Some device manufacturers recommend that the ClO_2-generating equipment remain outside the space being disinfected to prevent repeated exposure [34]. Instable in solution, chlorine dioxide must be mixed on-site by laboratory personnel. The effectiveness of ClO_2 in penetrating treated spaces may also cause concern for personnel safety, as it can migrate out of seemingly enclosed spaces [38, 40]. As a result, facilities employing ClO_2 systems must carefully monitor the disinfection cycle to ensure safety [64]. Roughly the size of an office bookcase and weighing approximately 230 pounds (104 kg), one system can treat up to 70,000 ft^3 (2,000 m^3) which may maximize the treatment space per device compared to other systems. ClO_2 can also be dispensed from smaller devices which fit into a biological safety cabinet to treat that equipment [67, 68].

4.3 High concentration H_2O_2 vapor

High concentration H_2O_2 devices are roughly the size of a medium file cabinet, wheeled around facilities on four castors and can be very heavy, weighing up to 500 pounds (227 kg). They are operated via touchscreen displays and the range of treatment area is between 8,800 to 20,000 ft^3 (249 to 566 m^3), depending on the device. One system can connect up to 10 devices via ethernet cables linking one device to another and enabling the treatment of larger spaces. Validation of these vaporous systems is determined using chemical and biological indicators, often *G. stearothermophilus* (1×10^6) an international standard for determining success in sterilization procedures [44]. These systems may not offer hand-spray or port-in capabilities; however, they can integrate into various chambers or rooms.

High concentration vaporous H_2O_2 systems traditionally employ a 35–59% H_2O_2 liquid solution, heated to a vaporous state [29]. These chemicals must be handled with care, since human contact with the liquid or vapor can be harmful and has been known to result in second- and third-degree burns [29–31]. Once heated, these chemicals are delivered to the treatment space, where vapor concentrations can reach peak levels of up to 1,400 ppm H_2O_2 [36], often necessitating precise operating conditions and continuous monitoring of the treatment cycle by the operator(s). A myriad of sensors precisely measures peak concentrations and these aid in delivering a specific combination of conditions to result in efficacy. These systems can be highly complex, accompanied by user manuals nearing a hundred pages of instructions. The four-part fogging process—dehumidification, conditioning, decontamination, and aeration—may require a technician to be present during the entire cycle of several hours [34, 69]. One reason for this vigilant monitoring may be to respond quickly should the system over or under deliver the high concentrations of H_2O_2 required. Another reason for persistent oversight may be a valid fear of escaped H_2O_2 vapor, which could migrate out of the treated space at high concentrations and affect personnel [38, 40].

4.4 Hydrogen peroxide silver ion devices

Chemical solutions, even within the range of H_2O_2 technologies, differ not only in concentration, but also in their formulation. Some available H_2O_2 solutions contain additional active ingredients, such as the heavy metal silver nitrate [70]. Although silver has a long history of use in wound care, it is also known to cause a permanent retention of silver once in the body [71]. Silver ions are one of the most toxic known forms of heavy metal [70]. Accidental ingestion of these invisible silver residues can cause problems for the microbiome of the human digestive system, since these metals lack the ability to differentiate beneficial bacteria from pathogenic bacteria [72]. Silver persists not only in the body, but also in the environment, where it remains toxic and can be lethal to organisms [70]. As a result of a growing understanding of these unintended negative consequences, the use of silver for disinfection is regulated by the European Union (BPR, Regulation (EU) 528/2012) which states that "It may unnecessarily expose humans, animals and the environment to biocidal active substance, generate health and/or environmental risks and impacts, and may also contribute to the development of resistance to biocides leading to other health and/or environmental issues" [73]. Likewise the EPA acknowledges the potential health hazards related to exposure to silver, and has issued cautionary documents to this effect [74]. Due to the high level of potential exposure during residue cleanup, and the resulting inhalation or dermal absorption of this heavy metal, proper protocols and control should be always employed [74]. Devices for aerosolizing H_2O_2 with silver vary in size from toolbox-sized fixed systems in mobile transportation to large, stand-alone portable systems. Some of these systems spray in a mist, while others use a more wet delivery method which may impede the generation of floating aerosols [75].

5. Key considerations when choosing a disinfection approach

There are several key elements to consider when deciding on a decontamination system. An ideal anti-microbial disinfectant should have the following characteristics: (1) is destructive to the greatest variety of pathogens, including bacterial spores, bacteria, viruses, molds, and fungi; (2) minimizes risks to personnel; (3) is non-corrosive and compatible with materials under normal application conditions; (4) is easy to implement; (5) imparts no harmful residue to the laboratory space or equipment; and (6) provides affordable decontamination. When comparing various disinfection systems, consider the most pertinent aspects below:

5.1 Highest efficacy

First and foremost, it is important for the system to not only be efficacious against more susceptible organisms, but efficacious against less susceptible organisms to the degree necessary to confidently implement the system as a regular component of the research cycle. Commensurate with the definitions of disinfection and decontamination [1], disinfection inactivates pathogens, while decontamination goes to the further degree of inactivating and denaturing them. In industries where pathogen-free environments form the foundational block for successful research, only decontamination will suffice. A detail-conscious manager should not only look for a decontaminant but select one which can demonstrate proof of efficacy with both porous and non-porous surfaces, most accurately representing the array found within life science sectors. Further supporting efficacy, laboratories should be able to validate their chosen system using biological indicators in adherence to international standards [44]. In support of risk management, the system should enable validation of sterilization through a 6-log_{10} sporicidal reduction that can be tracked and recorded [2]. With only the most efficacious systems under consideration, facility managers should evaluate each system's impact on personnel safety, ideal laboratory operation, equipment material compatibility, and integrity of research.

5.2 Safety

Even more important than the safety of materials is the safety of personnel, which should be a top priority when implementing a decontamination system. Safety should be considered from the perspective of normal operation as well as in the event of an accidental exposure. Under normal conditions, devices which can be operated remotely create a layer of isolation between the decontamination system and the human operator, allowing for implementation without direct contact for personnel. In the unlikely event of an accidental exposure, higher concentration solutions may come with risks for exposure to high-consequence chemicals either from contact or inhalation [39]. Choosing a product with lower operating concentrations may likewise decrease the potential for risks associated with accidental exposure caused by unintended fog leakage [38, 40]. As with most gaseous systems, the Occupational Safety and Health Administration (OSHA) has defined a minimum reoccupation level, Permissible Exposure Limit (PEL), which must be considered: ClO_2 = 0.1 ppm; H_2O_2 = 1 ppm; and formaldehyde = 0.75 ppm. Technologies employing lower operational ppm may reach reoccupation levels more quickly due to a lower peak threshold [15, 16, 76].

5.3 Consequences of repetitive use

Decontamination within facilities is a recurring need, so both the physical devices as well as the chemicals or solutions used in them should be reviewed for the consequences of regular use. Devices with instructions requiring the operating machinery to remain outside of the room being disinfected may call into question the safety of exposed laboratory equipment within this space [34]. Likewise, systems with operating concentrations that can condense at levels beyond known material compatibility, such as 45% hydrogen peroxide, may also damage laboratory equipment [33].

5.4 Ease of use

Decision makers should critically examine the number of parts necessary for implementing a system. Multiple components may appear to create value but instead may only introduce complication and risks. Hosing laying on the floor add contamination risk in two ways: (1) hoses may impede a complete disinfection of any surfaces they touch and (2) those same hoses may contribute to cross contamination as they are moved throughout the facility. Additionally, a system with many components also comes with many opportunities to misplace or damage a critical element, potentially disrupting scheduled disinfection cycles. Quality and durability of the equipment is paramount as well.

While not strictly required, the degree of support available also contributes to the ease of use of a system. Whether creating new protocols, training personnel, or troubleshooting unique challenges, ensuring there is a commitment from the vendor to provide support can mean the difference between a quick phone call or time spent deciphering a 100-page manual.

5.5 Residues

Besides providing ease of use, the optimal disinfectant will also be free of byproducts which can leave precipitates or residues behind on the treated surfaces, or damage those surfaces [56, 65, 73, 74]. Additives such as metals are often marketed as beneficial catalysts, yet any benefit imparted can be overshadowed by what is left behind. Any disinfection system should benefit the facility by controlling contaminants, rather than introducing them to sensitive laboratory environments. It is essential for the integrity of research that no residual components be left in a space perceived sterile which can interfere with, invalidate, or otherwise impact the scientific work taking place.

5.6 Costs

As cost-cutting measures within laboratory spaces continue to be important, one way to save money is to choose a system that can readily be operated in-house by personnel who feel safe doing so. Outsourcing can be associated with significantly higher costs. Systems that are safer, scalable, trackable, easy to use, and modular can be employed for more than one application, resulting in even more cost savings.

6. Conclusion

When striving to meet strict viral disinfection requirements yet achieve balance with ease of use, timeliness, and safety requirements, facility managers should assess the disinfection needs of individual laboratory environments and the facility as a whole. Ideal disinfection systems should include technologies that have the ability to achieve validated decontamination with the lowest risk to equipment and personnel. We believe that the Hybrid Hydrogen Peroxide system introduced and discussed in detail here merits consideration as a versatile tool for viral disinfection. Pulse technology provides an unexpected efficacy with a 7% H_2O_2 solution equaling the best commercially available high-concentration H_2O_2 systems. The simplicity of one portable device with optional accessories and integration capabilities offers intriguing possibilities for reaching and decontaminating viral pathogens that may be found in the myriad of spaces within laboratory environments. Although conceived with sterilization efficacy in mind, its simplicity of use and safer operation enabled widespread adoption into multiple markets such as education and the military, with applicators ranging from entry level technicians to experienced personnel. As research continues to venture into unknown territories, awareness of potential viral threats has increased as well. Current adoption into the life sciences field is robust and underscores the value which can be added through implementing a targeted yet versatile system for facility decontamination. This chapter provides encouragement that innovations in disinfection technology, such as the HHP system, continue to keep pace with these viral threats with fact-based, science-driven results.

Notes/thanks/other declarations

The authors would like to thank Jodi Woodson and Alyssa DeLotte for their invaluable contributions to this chapter.

Author details

Meaghan Hislop[1*], Frances Grinstead[1] and John R. Henneman[2]

1 CURIS System, Oviedo, FL, USA

2 Biosecurity Research Institute, Kansas State University, Manhattan, KS, USA

*Address all correspondence to: meg@curissystem.com

References

[1] Meechan P, Potts J. Biosafety in Microbiological and Biomedical Laboratories 6th Edition. U.S. Centers for Disease Control and Prevention (CDC); 2020. (CDC) 300859 https://www.cdc.gov/labs/pdf/SF__19_308133-A_BMBL6_00-BOOK-WEB-final-3.pdf. [Accessed: March 2021]

[2] U.S. Environmental Protection Agency (EPA) Office of Pesticide Programs. Protocol for Room Sterilization by Fogger Application. 2019. Available from: https://www.epa.gov/pesticide-registration/protocol-room-sterilization-fogger-application [Accessed: 2021-05-22]

[3] United States Environmental Protection Agency (EPA). Selected EPA-Registered Disinfectants. 2021. Available from: https://www.epa.gov/pesticide-registration/selected-epa-registered-disinfectants [Accessed: 2021-06-11]

[4] United States Environmental Protection Agency (EPA). Aerosol from Greenhouse Gas Emissions & Sinks Glossary Vocabulary Catalog. 1990-2002 [updated 2004 April 15; cited 2021 June 30]. Available from: https://search.epa.gov/epasearch/?querytext=Aerosol&areaname=&areacontacts=&areasearchurl=&typeofsearch=epa&result_template=2col.ftl#/

[5] Lexico. GAS: Definition of GAS in English by Oxford Dictionary. 2021. Available from: https://www.lexico.com/definition/Gas [Accessed: 2021-06-30]

[6] CURIS System. Comprehensive Hydrogen Peroxide Fogging. 2021. Available from: https://www.curissystem.com [Accessed: 2021-06-30]

[7] Lexico. Vapor: Definition of Vapor in English by Oxford Dictionary. 2021. Available from: https://www.lexico.com/en/definition/vapor [Accessed: 2021-06-30]

[8] Spaulding EH. Chemical disinfection of medical and surgical materials. In: Lawrence C, Block SS, editors. Disinfection, sterilization, and preservation. Philadelphia (PA): Lea & Febiger; 1968. p. 517–531.

[9] Sattar SA. Hierarchy of Susceptibility of Viruses to Environmental Surface Disinfectants: A Predictor of Activity Against New and Emerging Viral Pathogens. Journal of Association of Official Agricultural Chemists International 2007; 90:6:1655-1658. PMID: 18193744

[10] United States Environmental Protection Agency (EPA). What is an emerging viral pathogen claim? 2021. Available from: https://www.epa.gov/coronavirus/what-emerging-viral-pathogen-claim [Accessed: 2021-06-11]

[11] United States Environmental Protection Agency (EPA) Office of Pesticide Programs. Final Summary of the Disinfection Hierarchy Workshop. 2016. Available from: https://www.epa.gov/sites/production/files/2016-02/documents/dh_final_summary_of_workshop_-exploration_of_the_disinfection_hierarchy_meeting_summary_final_docx_2_4_16.pdf [Accessed: 2021-06-28]

[12] United States Environmental Protection Agency (EPA). Guidance to Registrants: Process for Making Claims Against Emerging Viral Pathogens Not on EPA-Registered Disinfectant Labels. 2016. Available from: https://www.epa.gov/sites/production/files/2016-09/documents/emerging_viral_pathogen_program_guidance_final_8_19_16_001_0.pdf [Accessed: 2021-06-30]

[13] Otter JA, Yezli S, Salkeld JA, French GL: Evidence that contaminated

surfaces contribute to the transmission of hospital pathogens and an overview of strategies to address contaminated surfaces in hospital settings. American Journal of Infection Control. 2013;41(5 Suppl):S6–11. 10.1016/j.ajic.2012.12.004

[14] United States Environmental Protection Agency (EPA). Compatibility of Material and Electronic Equipment with Hydrogen Peroxide and Chlorine Dioxide Fumigation. U.S. Environmental Protection Agency, Washington, DC, EPA/600/R-10/169, 2010.

[15] The National Institute for Occupational Safety and Health (NIOSH). Immediately Dangerous to Life or Health Concentrations (IDLH): Formaldehyde. U.S. Centers for Disease Control and Prevention (CDC); 1994 [updated: 2014-12-04]. Available from: https://www.cdc.gov/niosh/idlh/50000.html [Accessed: 2021-03-30]

[16] The National Institute for Occupational Safety and Health (NIOSH). Immediately Dangerous to Life or Health Concentrations (IDLH): Chlorine Dioxide. U.S. Centers for Disease Control and Prevention (CDC); 1994 [updated: 2004-12-04]. Available from: https://www.cdc.gov/niosh/idlh/10049044.html [Accessed: 2021-06-30]

[17] ClorDiSys Solutions: Safety Data Sheet Chlorine Dioxide Gas. SDS Code 50084. 2019. Available from: https://www.clordisys.com/pdfs/sds/SDS%20-%20Chlorine%20Dioxide%20Gas.pdf [Accessed: 2021-06-25]

[18] CURIS System: Safety Data Sheet CURoxideTM. 2021. Available from: https://www.curissystem.com/contact [Accessed: 2021-06-25]

[19] Derr H, James M, Kuny C, et al. Aerosolized Hydrogen Peroxide Decontamination of N95 Respirators, with Fit-Testing and Virologic Confirmation of Suitability for Re-Use During the COVID-19 Pandemic. medRXiV. DOI: https://doi.org/10.1101/2020.04.17.20068577

[20] Zarate V. GLP Custom Viricidal Whole Room Fogger Sterilization: Feline calicivirus (EPA approved human norovirus surrogate). 2020. Available from: https://www.curissystem.com [Accessed: 2021-03-30]

[21] Goyal SM, Chander Y, Yezli S, Otter JA. Evaluating the virucidal efficacy of hydrogen peroxide vapour. Jornal of Hospital Infection. 2014;86(4): 255-259. doi:10.1016/j.jhin.2014.02.003

[22] Heckert RA, Best M, Jordan LT, Dulac GC, Eddington DL, Sterritt WG. Efficacy of Vaporized Hydrogen Peroxide against Exotic Animal Viruses. Applied Environmental Microbiology [1997] p. 3916–3918. doi:10.1128/aem.63.10.3916-3918.

[23] Niethammer P, Grabher C, Look T, Mitchison T. A tissue-scale gradient of hydrogen peroxide mediates rapid wound detection in zebrafish. Nature. 2009 Jun 03 [cited 2021 June 25]; 459: 996-999. doi: 10.1038/nature08119

[24] Stock J, Stuart JD. The Decomposition of Hydrogen Peroxide by Blood. George Senter's Discovery of the Enzyme Involved. Bulletin for the History of Chemistry. 2005; 30:2

[25] Woodard, Curran. 7 Methods for Treating Wastewaters from Industry. In Woodard & Curran publishers. Industrial Waste Treatment Handbook 2nd edition. Butterworth-Heinemann. 2006. p. 149–334. https://doi.org/10.1016/B978-075067963-3/50009-6

[26] Melly E, Cowan AE, Setlow P. Studies on the mechanism of killing of Bacillus subtilis spores by hydrogen peroxide. Journal of Applied Microbiology. 2002; 93(2):316-325. doi: 10.1046/j.1365-2672.2002.01687.x. PMID: 12147081.

[27] IS Med Specialties. Hydrogen Peroxide Compatibility Chart Industrial Spec. 2020. Available from: https://www.industrialspec.com/images/files/hydrogen-peroxide-material-compatibility-chart-from-ism.pdf [Accessed: 2021-03-28]

[28] USP technologies. H2O2 Hazard Classes. 2021. Available from: https://www.h2o2.com/technical-library/default.aspx?pid=76&name=Hazard-Classes [Accessed: 2021-06-30]

[29] Peroxy Chem Safety Data Sheet Hydrogen Peroxide 35%; SDS No. 7722-84-1-35; PeroxyChem: Philadelphia, PA, 2015. https://www.h2o2.com/files/PeroxyChem_35_SDS.PDF [Accessed: 2021 June 30].

[30] Izu K, Yamamoto O, Asahi M. Occupational skin injury by hydrogen peroxide. Dermatology. 2000; 201(1): 61-64. DOI: 10.1159/000018434

[31] Shih S Y, Lai C C. Dermal Injury Caused by Hydrogen Peroxide. The Journal of Emergency Medicine. 2017; 53(6): 141–142. DOI: https://doi.org/10.1016/j.jemermed.2017.08.030

[32] Utah State University. Chapter 7: H2O2 Material Compatibility. Available from: http://mae-nas.eng.usu.edu/Peroxide_Web_Page/chapter_7.html [Accessed: 2021-06-30]

[33] Hultman C, Hill A, McDonnel G. The physical chemistry of decontamination with gaseous hydrogen peroxide. Pharmaceutical Engineering. 2007; 27(1): 22-32. Available from: https://static1.squarespace.com/static/52d6d893e4b0edcb252bf2af/t/52def125e4b0a28390ed4f61/1390342437903/Physical+Chemistry+of+Decon+with+Gaseous+H2O2.pdf

[34] Beswick A, Farrant J, Makison C, Gawn J, Frost G, Crook B, Pride J. Comparison of Multiple Systems for Laboratory Whole Room Fumigation. Applied Biosafafety. 2011; 16(3): 139-157. DOI: 10.1177/153567601101600303

[35] Principles of Chlorine Dioxide Gas as a Decontamination Method. Humidity's Role Towards Efficacy. ClorDiSys. Available from: https://www.clordisys.com/pdfs/conference/Kevin%20Lorcheim%20-%20Principles%20of%20CD%20Gas.pdf [Accessed: 2021-06-30]

[36] McAnoy AM, Sait M, Pantelidis S. Establishment of a Vaporous Hydrogen Peroxide Bio-Decontamination Capability. Australian Government Department of Defense, Defense Science and Technology Organization; 1994. DSTO-TR-1994. https://apps.dtic.mil/sti/pdfs/ADA470949.pdf [Accessed: 2021-08-25]

[37] Office of Chemical Safety and Pollution Prevention. CURoxide™ Master Label. United States Environmental Protection Agency (EPA). 2020. Available from: https://www3.epa.gov/pesticides/chem_search/ppls/093324-00001-20200716.pdf. [Accessed: 2021-05-30]

[38] Klostermyer J, Garcia A, Eddington D. Integrated Vapor-Phase Hydrogen Peroxide (VPHP) Decontamination Systems. 2017 Nov/Dec. Available from: https://ispe.org/pharmaceutical-engineering/november-december-2017/integrated-vapor-phase-hydrogen-peroxide-vphp# [Accessed: 2021-06-30]

[39] National Library of Medicine. Hydrogen Peroxide. Available from: https://webwiser.nlm.nih.gov/substance?substanceId=322&identifier=Hydrogen%20peroxide&identifierType=name&menuItemId=62&catId=83 [Accessed: 2021-06-30]

[40] ClorDiSys. Chlorine Dioxide Gas vs. Hydrogen Peroxide Vapor. Decontamination Penetration Issues.

ClorDiSys. Available from: https://www.clordisys.com/pdfs/ClorDiSysCDvsHPwebinar.pdf

[41] Henneman JR, McQuade EA, Sullivan RA, Downard J, Thackrah A, Hislop M. Analysis of Range and Use of a Hybrid Hydrogen Peroxide System for BSL-3 and ABSL Ag Laboratory Decontamination. Applied Biosafety. In press, 2021

[42] Ghidoni D, Grinstead F, Held K, Mullen R, Thibeault R. Effectiveness of aerosolized hydrogen peroxide in simultaneous decontamination of a laboratory and a biological safety cabinet. CURIS Company Publication. 2018. https://www.curissystem.com

[43] Thornley C, Emslie N, Sprott T, Greening G, Rapana J. Recurring norovirus transmission on an airplane. Clinical Infectious Diseases. 2011; 53(6): 515-520. DOI: 10.1093/cid/cir465.

[44] Kaspari O, Lemmer K, Becker S, et al. Decontamination of a BSL3 laboratory by hydrogen peroxide fumigation using three different surrogates for Bacillus anthracis spores. Journal of Applied Microbiology. 2014; 10.1111/jam.12601.

[45] Rutala W, Weber D, HICPAC. Guideline for Disinfection and Sterilization in Healthcare Facilities. Chapel Hill, NC: CDC; 2008 [updated: 2019-05; cited: 2021-06-26]. Available from: https://www.cdc.gov/infectioncontrol/pdf/guidelines/disinfection-guidelines-H.pdf

[46] Richard E. Evaluation of Surface Room Disinfection via Fogging Device Against *C. difficile*. MicroChem Laboratories GLP; 2019. Available from: https://www.curissystem.com [Accessed: 2021-03-28]

[47] Environmental Protection Agency (EPA). Consideration of Disinfection Hierarchy Concepts in the Registration of Antimicrobial Products. 2015. Available from: https://www.epa.gov/sites/default/files/2015-09/documents/disinfection-hierarchy-white-paper-draft.pdf [Accessed: 2021-06-30]

[48] National Collaborating Centre for Infectious Diseases. Norovirus. 2018. Available from: https://nccid.ca/debrief/norovirus/ [Accessed: 2021-06-20]

[49] Cirillo B. Containing an outbreak at the ground level: 100% decrease of non-enveloped virus norovirus in a 1500 bed assisted living facility. 2020. Available from: https://www.curissystem.com [Accessed: 2021-06-20]

[50] Goulding N. Antibacterial Activity and Efficacy of CURIS Bio-Decontamination's Liquid Disinfectant in Fogging Devices. MicroChem Laboratories GLP; 2021. Available from: https://www.curissystem.com [Accessed: 2021-06-20]

[51] Wibmann J E, Kirchhoff L, Bruggemann Y, et al. Persistence of pathogens on inanimate surfaces: a narrative review. Microorganisms. 2021; 9(2): 343. DOI: https://doi.org/10.3390/microorganisms9020343

[52] Centers for Disease Control and Prevention. Factors Affecting the Efficacy of Disinfection and Sterilization: Guideline for Disinfection and Sterilization in Healthcare Facilities. 2008. Available from: https://www.cdc.gov/infectioncontrol/guidelines/disinfection/efficacy.html [Accessed: 2021-06-30]

[53] United States Centers for Disease Control and Prevention (CDC). What is C. diff? 2020. Available from: https://www.cdc.gov/cdiff/what-is.html [Accessed: 2021-06-30]

[54] Rutala R, Kanamori H, Gergen M, et al. Enhanced disinfection leads to reduction of microbial contamination and a decrease in patient colonization

and infection. Infection Control Hospital Epidemiology. 2018; 39(9): 1118-1121. DOI: 10.1017/ice.2018.165

[55] Guideline for Disinfection and Sterilization in Healthcare Facilities. CDC. 2008. Available from: https://www.cdc.gov/infectioncontrol/guidelines/disinfection/disinfection-methods/chemical.html#Formaldehyde [Accessed: 2021-07-08]

[56] Ramage A. Fumigation of the Future. 2016. Available from: https://themedicinemaker.com/manufacture/fumigation-of-the-future [Accessed: 2021-07-08]

[57] Burrage S. Fumigation with Formaldehyde. Public Health Papers and Reports. 1897 [Accessed 2021-07-08]; 23: 110-113. Available from: https://www.ncbi.nlm.nih.gov/pmc/articles/PMC2329970/

[58] El Ashram M. The Use of Formaldehyde in Fumigation. EmTech Hatchery Systems. 2020. Available from: https://www.emtech-systems.com/technical-talk/the-use-of-formaldehyde-in-fumigation/ [Accessed: 2021-07-08]

[59] Thompson K. The Science of Disinfectants. CMM. 2012. Available from:https://www.cmmonline.com/articles/the-science-of-disinfectants [Accessed: 2021-07-08]

[60] Czarneski M. Selecting the Right Chemical Agent for Decontamination of Rooms and Chambers. Applied Biosafety. 2007; 12(2): 85-92. Available from: https://www.liebertpub.com/doi/pdfplus/10.1177/153567600701200204

[61] REACH. European Commission. Available from: https://ec.europa.eu/environment/chemicals/reach/reach_en.htm [Accessed: 2021-07-08]

[62] EPIZONE Workshop Formaldehyde Replacement. Lelystad, NL: Central Veterinary Institute; 2011 Jan. 32 p.

[63] Automated Formalin Preparation & Dispensing Device. Zenon. Available from: https://zenonmed.com/products/pathology/automated-formalin-preparation-dispensing-device/ [Accessed: 2021-07-08]

[64] Thermo Scientific Biological Safety Cabinets Fumigation Methodologies. Thermo Scientific. 2014. Available from: https://tools.thermofisher.com/content/sfs/brochures/BSC-Fumigation-Technical-Note.pdf [Accessed: 2021-07-08]

[65] Staschower F. Residues From Chlorine Dioxide Gas Treatment, Generated by Different Delivery Systems, on Fresh Produce [Master's Thesis]. Michigan State University; 2012. https://d.lib.msu.edu/etd/16 [Accessed: 2021-08-25]

[66] Principles of Chlorine Dioxide Gas as a Decontamination Method. Humidity's Role Towards Efficacy. ClorDiSys. Available from: https://www.clordisys.com/pdfs/conference/Kevin%20Lorcheim%20-%20Principles%20of%20CD%20Gas.pdf [Accessed: 2021-06-30]

[67] MINIDOX-M. ClorDiSys. 2014. Available from: https://www.clordisys.com/minidoxm.php [Accessed: 2021-07-08]

[68] Mini Chlorine Dioxide System (MCS). DRS Laboratories. Available from: http://drslaboratories.com/products/mini-chlorine-dioxide-system-mcs/ [Accessed: 2021-07-08]

[69] Kimura T, Yahata H, Uchiyama Y. Examination of Material Compatibilities with Ionized and Vaporized Hydrogen Peroxide Decontamination. Journal of the American Association for Laboratory Animal Science. 2020; 5(9): 703-711. DOI: 10.30802/AALAS-JAALAS-19-000165

[70] Ratte HT. Bioaccumulation and toxicity of silver compounds: A Review.

Environmental Toxicology and Chemistry. 2009; 18(1):89–108. DOI: https://doi.org/10.1002/etc.5620180112

[71] Lansdown AB. Silver in health care: antimicrobial effects and safety in use. Current Problems in Dermatology. 2006; 33:17-34.

[72] Li J, Tang M, Xue Y. Review of the effects of silver nanoparticle exposure on gut bacteria. Journal of Applied Toxicology. 2018; 39(1):27-37. DOI: https://doi.org/10.1002/jat.3729

[73] Culleen L, Fox T. No Silver Lining for Biocidal Products Now Under the EU Regulatory Cloud. Arnold & Porter; 2019 Oct 29. Available from: https://www.arnoldporter.com/en/perspectives/publications/2019/10/no-silver-lining-for-biocidal [Accessed: 2021-06-30]

[74] Davis M, Gillespie P, Gwinn M, Hendren C, Long T, Powers C. Nanomaterial Case Study: Nanoscale Silver in Disinfectant Spray. Research Triangle Park, NC: U.S. EPA; 2012 Aug. No. EPA/600/R-10/081F

[75] Sanosil. AEROSOL-TURBINE DEVICES. 2021. Available from: https://www.sanosil.com/en/product-lines/aerosoldisinfection/aerosol-turbine-devices/ [Accessed: 2021-07-08]

[76] The National Institute for Occupational Safety and Health (NIOSH). Immediately Dangerous to Life or Health Concentrations (IDLH): Hydrogen Peroxide. U.S. Centers for Disease Control and Prevention (CDC); 1994 [updated: 2014-12-04]. Available from: https://www.cdc.gov/niosh/idlh/772841.html [Accessed: 2021-03-30]

Chapter 4

Antiviral Coatings as Continuously Active Disinfectants

Luisa A. Ikner and Charles P. Gerba

Abstract

Antimicrobial surfaces and coatings have been available for many decades and have largely been designed to kill or prevent the growth of bacteria and fungi. Antiviral coatings have become of particular interest more recently during the COVID-19 pandemic as they are designed to act as continuously active disinfectants. The most studied antiviral coatings have been metal-based or are comprised of silane quaternary ammonium formulations. Copper and silver interact directly with proteins and nucleic acids, and influence the production of reactive free radicals. Titanium dioxide acts as a photocatalyst in the presence of water and oxygen to produce free radicals in the presence of UV light or visible light when alloyed with copper or silver. Silane quaternary ammonium formulations can be applied to surfaces using sprays or wipes, and are particularly effective against enveloped viruses. Continuously active disinfectants offer an extra barrier against fomite-mediated transmission of respiratory and enteric viruses to reduce exposure between routine disinfection and cleaning events. To take advantage of this technology, testing methods need to be standardized and the benefits quantified in terms of reduction of virus transmission.

Keywords: disinfection, virus, coating, continuously active, fomites

1. Introduction

Enteric and respiratory viruses can potentially be transmitted via contaminated environmental surfaces [1, 2]. Infectious viruses present on fomites may be transferred to the fingers and/or hands when touching various surface types under a broad spectrum of environmental conditions [3]. Transfer efficiency is affected by factors including virus species, inoculum size, and skin condition [4]. Subsequent contact with the eyes, nose, or mouth with contaminated fingers and hands may then provide access to susceptible human hosts [5]. Disinfection of environmental surfaces lowers the numbers of infectious microorganisms, thereby reducing the risk for transmission [6, 7]. However, such surfaces are subjected to continuous recontamination events, particularly in high-traffic areas and facilities including hospitals, daycare centers, schools and office buildings where fomites are more likely to serve as reservoirs of pathogens [8–10].

There are hundreds of liquid-based formulations that are registered as disinfectants with governmental regulatory agencies around the world, and a subset of those also carry label kill claims against non-enveloped and enveloped viruses. The efficacy testing that is required for the issuance of product label claims is performed using internationally-recognized standard test methods such as those produced by the American Standard for Test Materials (ASTM) and the European Standard (EN), among others. Liquid disinfectants can be applied to hard, non-porous surfaces using spray devices, towelettes (wipes), or as bulk liquid volumes to address large, soiled areas. To achieve the antiviral inactivation claims specified on product labels, disinfectants must be used according to the manufacturer's instructions which may require maintaining a completely wetted surface for up to 10 minutes. However, the habits and practices of product users are contrary to the directions specified on the label. A recent survey of American adults conducted on behalf of the American Cleaning Institute in 2020 revealed that 26% of respondents adhere to label directions during household disinfection routines; however, an equal percentage of those surveyed did profess to wiping surfaces until dry immediately after spraying with no adherence to contact time instructions [11]. An additional 16% of respondents claimed to use a single-pass method for disinfectant wipes rather than the multiple passes that are generally required to maintain surface wetness for several minutes.

The importance of correct disinfection usage has been of increased concern during the COVID-19 pandemic. Alternative disinfecting surface treatments that are capable of inactivating infectious agents, in particular viruses, are under research and development [12, 13]. A number of new and diverse antiviral coatings and films have been synthesized, and fixed or immobilized applications including solids (e.g., antimicrobial plastics), paints, and metals are increasingly of interest for their antiviral capabilities. The factors affecting virus survival and the efficacy of antiviral

Factor	Impact
Type of virus	Non-enveloped viruses are generally more resistant than enveloped viruses
Relative humidity	Drying rates of deposited viruses are affected, impacting viability
Temperature	Protein denaturation results in loss of structural integrity of virus
Soil (dirt) load	Increased demand on antiviral actives, decreasing availability for virus inactivation
Coating composition	Mechanisms of antiviral action differ among viruses and vary according to formulation
Contact Time	Time required for at least a 99.9% (3 $\log_{10}$) reduction in titer may range from minutes to hours

Table 1.
Factors that affect virus survival and efficacy of antiviral coatings [2, 14].

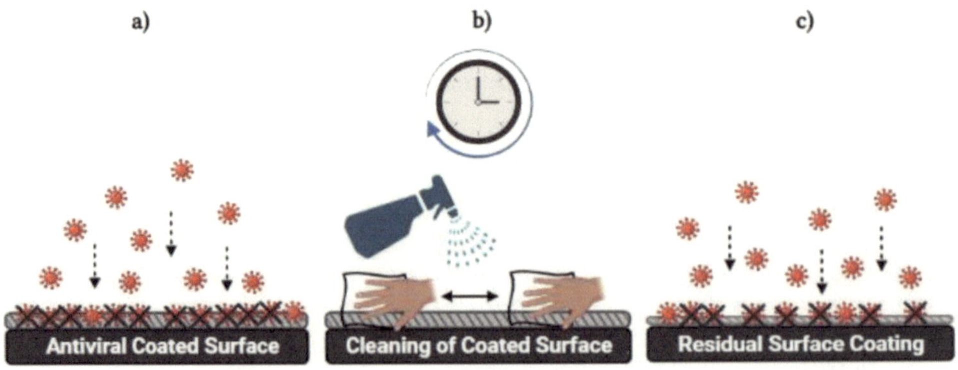

Figure 1.
Continuously active antiviral surface coatings: a) coating applied to hard, nonporous surface demonstrates antiviral activity following virus deposition; b) coated surfaces are cleaned/disinfected with wiping action with passage of time, c) residual coating demonstrates continuous antiviral efficacy following surface cleaning events (Created in BioRender.com).

coatings have been reviewed [2, 14] and include virus structure (i.e. enveloped, non-enveloped), the presence of organic soil (dirt), temperature, relative humidity, coating composition, and contact time (**Table 1**). The ability of treated surfaces to remain continuously active after repeated cleanings and use of liquid disinfectants is also critical (**Figure 1**). Unfortunately, there are no generally accepted methods for evaluating anti-viral surface coatings, making it difficult to compare the efficacy of different materials and studies. More research is warranted to better understand breadth of antiviral efficacy of these novel disinfecting technologies, and whether they can exact measurable and meaningful impacts on public health.

2. Continuously active disinfectants applied to hard, nonporous surfaces

A number of formulations have been developed and assessed over the past two decades that are capable of antiviral inactivation for extended periods of time following surface application (**Table 2**) [12–16]. Such applications have been considered as continuously active disinfectants and impart self-disinfecting properties to treated surfaces. There are many industry-based and third-party contract laboratory studies that have evaluated the antiviral properties of these surface treatments. However, few have been published to-date in peer-reviewed scientific journals [17], with an even smaller subgroup assessing efficacy against infectious viral agents. Continuously active disinfectants are generally evaluated for residual inactivation efficacy using a controlled, standardized wear and abrasion procedure such as that described in United States EPA Protocol #01-1A [18]. Briefly, a product applied to a hard non-porous surface is subjected to alternating dry and moistened wiping procedures over a specified time period (≥ 24 hours) with intermittent reinoculations of the test organism. A minimum of 12 wear cycles is required, and the remaining film of test product is challenged by a final dose of the target organism (≥ 4.8 $\log_{10}$) for up to 5 minutes of contact time. Residual efficacy depends in part on the amount of disinfectant remaining on the surface after the wear and abrasion testing which indicates its durability. Products that are readily removed from surfaces during repeated wet and dry wiping events could require regular reapplication to ensure proper performance against target microbes. As with standard disinfection,

Coating*	Type of viruses tested against†,‡	Mechanism of inactivation
Silane polymer QAC	Influenza, HCoV-229E, SARS-CoV-2, feline calicivirus	Behaves as a surfactant; disrupts lipid and protein structure
Copper	Influenza A, hepatitis A, feline calicivirus, adenovirus, HCoV- 229E, SARS-CoV2	Reactive oxygen species; protein and nucleic acid denaturization
Silver	Influenza, SARS-CoV2, HCoV-229E, murine norovirus	Reaction with sulfhydryl groups in proteins; prevention of viral attachment to host cells
Zinc	Murine norovirus, SARS-CoV-2, influenza	Inhibiting proteolytic cleavage, preventing synthesis of viral polypeptides
Titanium dioxide	Influenza, adenovirus; SARS-Co-2	Generation of reactive hydroxyl radicals

**QAC: quaternary ammonium compound.*
†HCoV-229E: human coronavirus 229E.
‡SARS-CoV-2: SARS-related coronavirus 2.

Table 2.
Common antiviral surface chemistries and mechanisms of action [12–16].

residual effectiveness generally follows the hierarchy of susceptibility of viruses to disinfectants, where enveloped viruses are more susceptible to inactivation than non-enveloped viruses [19].

Quaternary ammonium compounds (QAC) have been in general use by industry and consumers for almost 70 years, mostly as rapid-action ($\leq$ 10 minutes contact time) spray disinfectants for contaminated surfaces. They are considered as cationic surfactants or detergents, and are highly effective at disrupting the inner membranes of bacteria and lipid bilayers of enveloped viruses. QAC have undergone formulation changes to enhance effectiveness against non-enveloped viruses [20]. When combined with silane and polymers, they can be applied as a surface coating with antimicrobial properties [21]. Silane-QAC are long-chain molecules comprised of three principal components: 1) a silane base for covalent bonding to surfaces; 2) a centrally-located positively-charged nitrogen component, and 3) a long chain 'spear' consisting of a methyl hydrocarbon group. They can be applied to hard surfaces and to fabrics, and their virucidal efficacies may persist from 24 hours to weeks on treated surfaces.

Peer-reviewed studies evaluating the effectiveness of QAC-based surface coating treatments against viruses are currently limited. A quaternary ammonium polymer coating applied to stainless steel coupons demonstrated greater than 99.9% (>3 $\log_{10}$) reduction during 2 hours of contact against SARS-CoV-2 and human coronavirus 229E in the presence of 5% organic soil, although wear testing was not performed to assess residual antiviral activity [22]. Another study evaluating a QAC applied onto acrylic surfaces against subsequent SARS-CoV-2 and human coronavirus 229E contamination events demonstrated rapid inactivation upon contact (>90% [>1 $\log_{10}$] reduction); however, just one cleaning event of the coating using a water-based detergent and microfiber cloth substantially reduced product efficacy [23]. More peer-reviewed research is needed to better understand the breadth of QAC coating efficacy against the spectrum of non-enveloped and enveloped viruses, and under varying soil load and environmental conditions. Additional studies are also warranted to assess the durability of these coatings following simulated touches and cleaning events, and the resulting impacts on antiviral effectiveness.

3. Titanium dioxide

Titanium dioxide (TiO_2) is a photocatalytic inorganic chemistry that can be applied to a wide variety of surface types to provide antiviral protection. It does not inactivate viruses directly, but acts as a catalyst in the presence of UVA light (wavelength 315 to 400 nm) to generate reactive oxygen species that cause structural damage to viruses. The presence of moisture (in the air or on the surface) and oxygen are necessary for TiO_2 to be an effective antiviral agent. Light intensity is also key in driving the photocatalytic reaction. Residual photocatalytic activity may also occur in the dark after exposure to UV light, but is dependent on the prior exposure intensity.

Most of the studies evaluating the antimicrobial effectiveness of TiO_2 have focused on bacteria, and data on viruses remains scant in the literature [16]. TiO_2 has demonstrated >3 $\log_{10}$ reduction against influenza A within 4 hours, and > 1 $\log_{10}$ inactivation of feline calicivirus within 8 hours [24]. TiO_2 coatings have also been modified with fluorine to increase the production of reactive oxygen species under the low UVA-intensity fluorescent lighting that is typically found within indoor settings. Bacteriophage MS2, feline calicivirus, and murine norovirus infectivity levels were reduced by 2.6, 2.0, and 2.6 $\log_{10}$, respectively, on fluorinated TiO_2

surfaces [25]. The antiviral action of TiO_2 can be further enhanced within indoor environments by the addition of metals [26, 27]. A 1% silver-amended TiO_2 formulation yielded >4.00 log_{10} reduction of influenza A and enterovirus following a 20-minute exposure in the presence of a low intensity (15 W) UVA lamp [28]. More recently, infectious SARS-CoV-2 was reduced to levels below detection on TiO_2 and TiO_2-Silver (Ag) ceramic-coated tiles within 5 hours of exposure [15].

4. Metals

Metals such as copper, silver, and gold have been recognized since ancient times as having some health benefits, and the antibacterial properties of metals have since been well-studied [29]. In contrast, the mechanisms of metal inactivation of specific viruses remain unclear, although a number have been proposed and evaluated. Certain metals in trace amounts are critical to the function of viral proteins and genetic processes; however, levels in excess cause structural damage and affect viability [14]. The presence of these metals stimulates the generation of reactive oxygen species and damages viral envelopes as well as nucleocapsid proteins [30]. Metals can be incorporated into plastics and fabrics, used as actives in coating formulations, and fashioned directly into surfaces for direct use (e.g., copper sheets for incorporation into high-touch surfaces).

4.1 Copper

The antimicrobial properties of copper have been extensively studied, with efficacy demonstrated over a broad range of temperature and humidity values [1]. The proposed antiviral mechanisms of solid-state copper, copper oxides, and copper alloys against enveloped and non-enveloped viruses have been thoroughly reviewed [31]. Copper (I), (II), (III) ions act directly by denaturing viral surface proteins, and indirectly by the formation of reactive oxygen species that damage viral RNA and DNA. Copper surfaces inactivated infectious influenza A (H1N1) within 6 hours by 3 to 4 log_{10}, relative to virus levels remaining on stainless steel coupons [32]. Although copper has demonstrated broad-spectrum antimicrobial activity, it may be impractical to replace bulk materials within high-traffic areas (e.g., clinical settings) with copper products or components. The recent development of cold- and thermally-applied copper sprays, as well as fixed copper nanoparticle coatings and paints, enables continuously active disinfection measures against a spectrum of viruses [16]. Copper nanoparticles in the oxide form have shown promise against herpes simplex virus, human norovirus, and influenza A (H1N1) [31]. When applied using the cold spray technique, copper nanoparticles reduced infectious influenza A virus particles to levels below detection within 10 minutes [33].

4.2 Silver

The antimicrobial properties of silver have been known for more than a century. Much of the research investigating the antimicrobial properties of silver has examined inactivation in suspension, where lower doses are required to achieve inactivation effects relative to other metals [34]. Silver binds with disulfide (S-S) and sulfhydryl (-SH) groups in proteins, facilitates the production of reactive oxygen species (e.g., free radicals), and is believed to inhibit entry of HIV-1 into CD4+ host cells [35]. Unlike copper, the efficacy of silver decreases markedly at relative humidity levels <20% [1], and solid-state silver appears to be much less effective against bacteriophage Qβ and influenza A than solid-state copper [36]. For surface applications, silver nanoparticles have been extensively researched. Silver nitrate and silver nanoparticles in surface coatings reduced recoverable levels of feline calicivirus and murine norovirus for up to 150 days [37]. Silver has also been incorporated into fabrics (hospital gowns, pillowcases, cotton sheets), textiles, and membranes, demonstrating antiviral properties against feline calicivirus and murine norovirus, as well as enveloped viruses [16, 38].

4.3 Zinc

The antiviral properties of zinc have been researched for the past several decades. Zinc inhibits proteolytic cleavage and the synthesis of viral polypeptides by human rhinovirus [39], and interferes with polymerase function and protein production by herpes simplex virus 1 [16]. For surface applications, pure zinc, itself, does not exhibit high levels of antiviral activity. A 1 $\log_{10}$ reduction of murine norovirus on pure zinc was measured within 2 hours, relative to complete inactivation of the test virus via synergism when exposed to a copper-silver-zinc alloy [40]. On plastic coupons with incorporated silver/copper-zeolites, >1.7 $\log_{10}$ and > 3.8 $\log_{10}$ reductions were achieved for human coronavirus 229E and feline calicivirus, respectively, within 24 hours [41]. More recently, zinc ion-embedded polyamide fibers were found to reduce levels of infectious influenza A and SARS-CoV-2 by approximately 2 $\log_{10}$ within 30 minutes [42].

5. Novel antiviral surface treatments

Research efforts are ongoing for the development of novel and continuously active coatings that are capable of maintaining low levels of bioburden while inactivating pathogenic microorganisms. A thorough review has been published of these coatings and their proposed mechanisms of action [14, 43]. The antiviral actives include biopolymers (e.g., antimicrobial peptides), synthetic polymers (e.g., polyethyleneimines, and graphene [14, 44, 45]. Natural product-based surface coatings and super-hydrophobic surfaces are also under development [46, 47]. Although many of these innovative technologies demonstrate promising antiviral effectiveness, further assessments of efficacy against additional types of viruses under various conditions are required. Reproducibility data generated among different lab groups would also be ideal to ensure product efficacy and reliability. Further, scaling up from the lab bench to assess these technologies under real-world conditions (i.e. placement into high-traffic, high-touch areas) will provide insight as to the consistency of their efficacy.

6. Conclusions and recommendations

From this review, it is clear that promising antiviral continuously active disinfectants are a reality. However, many obstacles exist before their widespread implementation. These include:

- Development and validation of standard methods for testing the efficacy of antiviral continuously active disinfectants. Ideally, these methods would indicate appropriate experimental conditions including relative humidity and temperature, organic soil load matrices, and evaluation of virucidal efficacy against enveloped and non-enveloped viruses.

- Establishing an acceptable contact time for a 3 $\log_{10}$ (99.9%) decrease in infectious virus. Some continuously active disinfectants can achieve this goal within a few minutes, and others may require 1 to 2 hours.

- Demonstration of the reduction in illnesses within facilities in which continuously active disinfectants are used. This is an ideal requirement, but difficult to achieve because of the high cost and multiple routes by which enteric and respiratory viruses can be transmitted. Reductions in hospital-acquired infections have been demonstrated with the use of copper [48–49] and silane QAC [50] disinfectants, but such studies are not always ideal because of limitations inherent in epidemiological studies, and extracting precision is usually lacking. Further, more information is needed as to the potential human health and environmental impacts of silane QAC usage in these settings.

- Application of quantitative microbial risk assessment (QMRA) to quantify the cost/benefits of continuously active disinfectants. QMRA is a lower-cost approach to documenting the probability of disease reduction that can be achieved. It can be used to estimate the difference in benefits from a continuously active disinfectant that inactivates 99.9% of the virus within 1 minute vs. one that achieves this within 2 hours.

- Education of regulators, public health officials, and the general public is necessary to ultimately achieve the benefits of continuously active disinfectants. There is concern that their use may provide a false sense of security, causing consumers to clean and disinfect less frequently. Continuously active disinfectants should be looked upon as an additional barrier, and not as a replacement for routine cleaning and disinfection.

Conflict of interest

The authors have no conflict of interest to declare.

Author details

Luisa A. Ikner* and Charles P. Gerba
Department of Environmental Science, The University of Arizona, Tucson, AZ, United States of America

*Address all correspondence to: ikner@arizona.edu

References

[1] Castaño N, Cordts S, Kurosu Jalil M, Zhang K, Koppaka S, Bick A, et al. Fomite transmission, physicochemical origin of virus–surface interactions, and disinfection strategies for enveloped viruses with applications to SARS-CoV-2. ACS Omega. 2021;**6**:6509-6527. DOI: 10.1021/acsomega.0c06335

[2] Boone S, Gerba C. Significance of fomites in the spread of respiratory and enteric viral disease. Applied and Environmental Microbiology. 2007; **73**:1687-1696. DOI: 10.1128/AEM.02051-06

[3] Lopez G, Gerba C, Tamimi A, Kitajima M, Maxwell S, Rose J. Transfer efficiency of bacteria and viruses from porous and nonporous fomites to fingers under different relative humidity conditions. Applied and Environmental Microbiology. 2013;**79**:5728-5734. DOI: 10.1128/AEM.01030-13

[4] Julian T, Leckie J, Boehm A. Virus transfer between fingerpads and fomites. Journal of Applied Microbiology. 2010;**109**:1868-1874. DOI: 10.1111/j.1365-2672.2010.04814.x

[5] Nicas M, Best D. A study quantifying the hand-to-face contact rate and its potential application to predicting respiratory tract infection. Journal of Occupational and Environmental Hygiene. 2008;**5**:347-352. DOI: 10.1080/15459620802003896

[6] Rutala W, Kanamori H, Gergen M, Knelson L, Sickbert-Bennett E, Chen L, et al. CDC prevention epicenters program Enhanced disinfection leads to reduction of microbial contamination and a decrease in patient colonization and infection. Infection Control & Hospital Epidemiology. 2018;**39**:1118-1121. DOI: 10.1017/ice.2018.165

[7] Rutala W, Weber D. The benefits of surface disinfection. American Journal of Infection Control. 2004;**32**:226-231

[8] Kraay A, Hayashi M, Berendes D, Sobolik J, Leon J, Loopman B. Risk for fomite-mediated transmission of SARS-CoV-2 in child daycares, schools, and nursing homes, and offices. Emerging Infectious Diseases. 2021; **27**:1229-1231. DOI: 10.3201/eid2704.203631

[9] Weber D, Anderson D, Rutala W. The role of the surface environment in healthcare-associated infections. Current Opinion in Infectious Diseases. 2013;**26**:338-344. DOI: 10.1097/QCO.0b013e3283630f04

[10] Hardy K, Gossain S, Henderson N, Drugan C, Oppenheim B, Gao F, et al. Rapid recontamination with MRSA of the environment of an intensive care unit after decontamination with hydrogen peroxide vapour. Journal of Hospital Infection. 2007;**66**:360-368. DOI: 10.1016/j.jhin.2007.05.009

[11] The American Cleaning Institute. Cleaning and COVID-19: Survey Shows 42% not disinfecting properly [Internet]. 2020. Available from: https://www.cleaninginstitute.org/newsroom/releases/cleaning-and-covid-19-survey [Accessed: October 21, 2021]

[12] Kumari S, Chatterjee K. Biomaterials-based formulations and surfaces to combat viral infectious diseases. APL Bioengineering. 2021;**5**:011503. DOI: 10.1063/5.0029486

[13] Shirvanimoghaddam K, Skbari M, Yadav R, Al-Tamimi A, Naebe M. Fight against COVID-19: The case of antiviral surfaces. APL Materials. 2021;**9**:031112. DOI: 10.1063/5.0043009

[14] Rakowska P, Tiddia M, Faruqui N, Bankier C, Pei Y, Pollard A, et al. Antiviral surfaces and coatings and their mechanisms of action. Communications Materials. 2021;**2**:1-19. DOI: 10.1038/s43246-021-00153-y

[15] Micochova P, Chadha A, Hesseloj T, Fraternali F, Ramsden J, Gupta R. Rapid inactivation of SARS-CoV-2 by titanium dioxide surface coating. Wellcome Open Research. 2021;**6**:56. DOI: 10.12688/wellcomeopenres.16577.1

[16] Imani S, Ladouceur L, Marshall T, Maclachlan R, Soleymani L, Didar T. Antimicrobial nanomaterials and coatings: Current mechanisms and future perspectives to control the spread of viruses including SARS-CoV-2. ACS Nano. 2020;**14**:12341-12369. DOI: 10.1021/acsnano.0c05937

[17] Rutala W, Gergen W, Sickbert-Bennett E, Anderson D, Weber D. Antimicrobial activity of a continuously active disinfectant against healthcare pathogens. Infection Control & Hospital Epidemiology. 2019;**40**:1284-1286. DOI: 10.1017/ice.2019.260

[18] United States Environmental Protection Agency. Protocol for Residual Self-Sanitizing Activity of Dried Chemical Residues on Hard, Non-Porous Surfaces: #01-1A. Washington D.C., United States: United States Environmental Protection Agency. 2015. Available from: https://www.epa.gov/sites/production/files/2015-09/documents/cloroxpcol_final.pdf [Accessed: February 16, 2016]

[19] Sattar S. Hierarchy of susceptibility of viruses to environmental surface disinfectants: A predictor of activity against new and emerging viral pathogens. Journal of AOAC International. 2007;**90**:1655-1658. DOI: 10.1093/jaoac/90.6.1655

[20] Gerba C. Quaternary ammonium biocides: Efficacy in application. Applied and Environmental Microbiology. 2015;**81**:464-469. DOI: 10.1128/AEM.02633-14

[21] McDonnell G. Antisepsis, Disinfection and Sterilization. 2nd ed. Washington, DC: ASM Press; 2017. p. 410

[22] Ikner L, Torrey J, Gundy P, Gerba C. Efficacy of an antiviral surface coating against human coronavirus 229E and SARS-CoV-2. American Journal of Infection Control. 2021;**49**(12):1569-1571. DOI: 10.1016/j.ajic.2021.08.031

[23] Butot S, Baert L, Zuber S. Assessment of antiviral coatings for high-touch surfaces by using human coronaviruses HCoV-229E and SARS-CoV-2. Applied and Environmental Microbiology. 2021;**87**:e01098-e01021. DOI: 10.1128/AEM.01098-21

[24] Nakano R, Hara M, Ishiguro H, Yao Y, Ochiai T, Nakata K, et al. Broad spectrum microbicidal activity of photocatalysis by TiO2. Catalysts. 2013;**3**:310-323. DOI: 10.3390/catal3010310

[25] Park G, Cho M, Cates E, Lee D, Oh B, Vinjé J, et al. Fluorinated TiO2 as an ambient light-activated virucidal surface coating material for the control of human norovirus. Journal of Photochemistry and Photobiology B: Biology. 2014;**140**:315-320. DOI: 10.1016/j.jphotobiol.2014.08.009

[26] Miyauchi M, Sunada K, Hashimoto K. Antiviral effect of visible light-sensitive CuxO/TiO2 photocatalyst. Catalysts. 2020;**10**:1093. DOI: 10.3390/catal10091093

[27] Moongraksathum B, Chien M, Chen Y. Antiviral and antibacterial effects of silver-doped TiO2 prepared by the peroxo sol-gel method. Journal of Nanoscience and Nanotechnology. 2019;**19**:7356-7362. DOI: 10.1166/jnn.2019.16615

[28] Liu M, Sunada K, Miyauchi HK. Visible-light sensitive Cu(II)-TiO2 with sustained anti-viral activity for efficient indoor environmental remediation. Journal of Materials Chemistry A. 2015;**3**:17312-17319. DOI: 10.1039/C5TA03756E

[29] Lemire J, Harrison J, Turner R. Antimicrobial activity of metals: Mechanisms, molecular targets and applications. Nature Reviews Microbiology. 2013;**11**:371-384. DOI: 10.1038/nrmicro3028

[30] Sunada K, Minoshima M, Hashimoto K. Highly efficient antiviral and antibacterial activities of solid-state cuprous compounds. Journal of Hazardous Materials. 2021;**235**:265-270. DOI: 10.1016/j.jhazmat.2012.07.052

[31] Govind V, Bharadwaj S, Sai Ganesh M, Vishnu J, Shankar K, Shankar B, et al. Antiviral properties of copper and its alloys to inactivate covid-19 virus: A review. Biometals. 2021;**34**:1-19. DOI: 10.1007/s10534-021-00339-4

[32] Noyce J, Michels H, Keevil C. Inactivation of influenza A virus on copper versus stainless steel surfaces. Applied and Environmental Microbiology. 2007;**73**:2748-2750. DOI: 10.1128/AEM.01139-06

[33] Champagne V, Sundberg K, Helfritch D. Kinetically deposited copper antimicrobial surfaces. Coatings. 2019;**9**:257. DOI: 10.3390/coatings 9040257

[34] Silvestry-Rodriguez N, Sicarios-Ruelas K, Gerba C, Bright K. Silver as a disinfectant. Reviews of Environmental Contamination and Toxicology. 2007;**191**:23-45. DOI: 10.1007/978-0-387-69163-3_2

[35] Lara H, Ayala-Nuñez N, Ixtepan-Turrent L, Rodriguez-Padilla C. Mode of antiviral action of silver nanoparticles against HIV-1. Journal of Nanobiotechnology. 2010;**8**:1-10. DOI: 10.1186/1477-3155-8-1

[36] Minoshima M, Lu Y, Kimura T, Nakano R, Ishiguro H, Kubota Y, et al. Comparison of the antiviral effect of solid-state copper and silver compounds. Journal of Hazardous Materials. 2016;**312**:1-7. DOI: 10.1016/j.jhazmat.2016.03.023

[37] Castro-Mayorga J, Randazzo W, Fabra M, Lagaron J, Aznar R, Sanchez G. Antiviral properties of silver nanoparticles against norovirus surrogates and their efficacy in coated polyhyroyalkanoates systems. LWT – Food Science and Technology. 2017;**79**:503-510. DOI: 10.1016/j.lwt.2017.01.065

[38] Gerba C, Sifuentes L, Lopez G, Abd-Elmaksound S, Calabrese J, Tanner B. Wide-spectrum activity of a silver-impregnated fabric. American Journal of Infection Control. 2016;**44**:689-690. DOI: 10.1016/j.ajic.2015.11.033

[39] Korant B, Kauer J, Butterworth B. Zinc ions inhibit replication of rhinoviruses. Nature. 1974;**248**:588-590. DOI: 10.1038/248588a0

[40] Warnes S, Summersgill E, Keevil C. Inactivation of murine norovirus on a range of copper surfaces is accomplished by a loss of capsid integrity. Applied and Environmental Microbiology. 2015;**81**:1085-1091. DOI: 10.1128/AEM.03280-14

[41] Bright K, Sicarios-Ruelas E, Gundy P, Gerba C. Assessment of the antiviral properties of zeolites containing metal ions. Food and Environmental Virology. 2008;**1**:37-41. DOI: 10.1007/s12560-008-9006-1

[42] Gopal V, Nilsson-Payant B, French H, Siegers J, Yung W, Hardwick M, et al. Zinc-embedded polyamide fabrics inactivate SARS-CoV-2 and influenza A virus. ACS Applied Materials & Interfaces. 2021;**13**:30317-30325. DOI: 10.1021/acsami.1c04412

[43] Bäumler W, Eckl D, Holzmann T, Schneider-Brachert W. Antimicrobial

coatings for environmental surfaces in hospitals: A potential new pillar for prevention strategies in hygiene. Critical Reviews in Microbiology. 2021:1-35. DOI: 10.1080/1040841X.2021.1991271

[44] Reina G, Iglesias D, Samorì P, Bianco A. Graphene: A disruptive opportunity for COVID-19 and future pandemics? Advanced Materials. 2021;*33*:2007847. DOI: 10.1002/adma.202007847

[45] Basak S, Packirisamy G. Nano-based antiviral coatings to combat viral infections. Nano-Structures & Nano-Objects. 2020;**24**:100620. DOI: 10.1016/j.nanoso.2020.100620

[46] Chauhan P, Kumar A. Development of a microbial coating for cellulosic surface using aloe vera and silane. Carbohydrate Polymer Technologies and Applications. 2020;**1**:100015. DOI: 10.1016/j.carpta.2020.100015

[47] Elzaabalawy A, Meguid S. Potential of combating transmission of COVID-19 using novel self-cleaning superhydrophobic surfaces: Part II—thermal, chemical, and mechanical durability. International Journal of Mechanics and Materials in Design. 2020;**16**:433-441. DOI: 10.1007/s10999-020-09512-y

[48] Michels H, Keevil C, Salgado C, Schmidt M. From laboratory research to a clinical trial: Copper alloy surfaces kill bacteria and reduce hospital-acquired infections. HERD: Health Environments Research & Design Journal. 2015;**9**:64-79. DOI: 10.1177/1937586715592650

[49] Salgado C, Sepkowitz K, John J, Cantey J, Attaway H, Freeman K, et al. Copper surfaces reduce the rate of healthcare-acquired infections in the intensive care unit. Infection Control & Hospital Epidemiology. 2013;**34**:479-486. DOI: 10.1086/670207

[50] Ellingson K, Pogreba-Brown K, Gerba C, Elliott S. Impact of a novel antimicrobial surface coating on health care–associated infections and environmental bioburden at 2 urban hospitals. Clinical Infectious Diseases. 2020;**71**:1807-1813. DOI: 10.1093/cid/ciz1077

Chapter 5

Predicted and Measured Virucidal Efficacies of Microbicides for Emerging and Re-emerging Viruses Associated with WHO Priority Diseases

M. Khalid Ijaz, Raymond W. Nims, Todd A. Cutts, Julie McKinney and Charles P. Gerba

Abstract

The World Health Organization has updated its list of priority diseases for 2021 to currently include the following: Ebola virus disease and Marburg virus disease (*Filoviridae*), Nipah and henipaviral diseases (*Paramyxoviridae*), Lassa fever (*Arenaviridae*), Rift Valley fever and Crimean-Congo hemorrhagic fever (*Bunyaviridae*), Zika (*Flaviviridae*), COVID-19 (SARS-CoV-2) including Delta, Omicron, and other variants of concern, Middle East respiratory syndrome, severe acute respiratory syndrome (*Coronaviridae*), and the always present "disease X," which is a term used for the next emerging pathogen of concern that is not known about today. In this chapter, we review the virucidal efficacy data for microbicides (*disinfectants and antiseptics, also known as surface and hand hygiene agents or collectively hygiene agents*) for the viruses associated with these diseases. As these diseases are each caused by lipid-enveloped viruses, the susceptibilities of the viruses to virucidal agents are informed by the known hierarchy of susceptibility of pathogens to microbicides. The unique susceptibility of lipid-enveloped viruses to most classes of microbicides is based on the common mechanism of action of envelope-disrupting microbicides. Empirical data supporting this principle and the mitigational role of targeted hygiene in infection prevention and control (IPAC) discussed are presented.

Keywords: Coronaviruses, Crimean-Congo hemorrhagic fever virus, Ebola virus, Lassa virus, Marburg virus, MERS-CoV, Nipah virus, Rift Valley fever virus, SARS-CoV, SARS-CoV-2, virus inactivation, Zika virus

1. Introduction

The World Health Organization (WHO) compiles, each year, a list of priority diseases. As stated in the associated WHO web page [1], the list is intended to encourage "research and development in emergency contexts." In other words, recognizing that the number of pathogens is very large, the WHO attempts through the Priority List to focus research attention on those diseases posing the greatest risk to public health. In addition, the Priority List serves to promote the development of infection prevention and control (IPAC) "countermeasures" for diseases where such countermeasures are limited or non-existent [1].

In this chapter, we thought it would be of interest to examine the 2021 WHO Priority List (**Box 1**) to see where the public health community stands with respect to IPAC countermeasures for the listed viruses (see section below). The approach that we have taken involved searching the literature for articles pertaining to virucidal efficacies for microbicides evaluated specifically against the listed viruses. In some cases literature for a specific listed virus was not able to be identified, but literature on listed viruses of the same family were available. The mechanisms of action of microbicides for viruses should apply similarly to different members of a given virus family, although intrafamily exceptions do exist [2, 3].

The WHO priority diseases [1] are updated periodically in "a list of disease and pathogens [that is] prioritized for R&D in public health emergency contexts." This tool specifies "which diseases pose the greatest public health risk due to their epidemic potential and/or whether there is no or insufficient countermeasures."

At present, the priority diseases are:

- COVID-19 [SARS-CoV-2, including its variants]
- Crimean-Congo haemorrhagic fever
- Ebola virus disease and Marburg virus disease
- Lassa fever
- Middle East respiratory syndrome coronavirus (MERS-CoV) and Severe Acute Respiratory Syndrome (SARS)
- Nipah and henipaviral diseases
- Rift Valley fever
- Zika
- "Disease X"*

*Disease X represents the knowledge that a serious international epidemic could be caused by a pathogen currently unknown to cause human disease [1].

Box 1.
WHO priority disease list.

It should be noted, as a starting point, that even in the absence of empirical data supporting the virucidal efficacy of microbicides for a given emerging or re-emerging virus or mutational variant of a known virus such as emerging variants of SARS-CoV-2, disinfection options still are available for IPAC. For instance, the United States Environmental Protection Agency (U.S. EPA) has invoked an Emerging Viral Pathogen Guidance for Antimicrobial Pesticides [4, 5] specifically to deal with just such a possibility. As stated in the associated U.S. EPA web page, the guidance provides a "process that can be used to identify effective disinfectant products for use against emerging viral pathogens and to permit registrants to make limited claims of their product's efficacy against such pathogens." The actual guidance (Guidance to Registrants: Process for Making Claims against Emerging Viral Pathogens not on EPA-registered Disinfectant Labels) [5] outlines "a voluntary two stage process, involving product label amendments and modified terms of registration and applies only to emerging viruses" [4].

The underlying principle driving the U.S. EPA Guidance for Antimicrobial Pesticides is that of the hierarchy of susceptibility of pathogens to microbicides (the so-called Spaulding Classification [6]). In the U.S. EPA guidance [5], viruses are classified into three categories, ranked from lesser to greater susceptibility to microbicides: small, non-enveloped viruses; large, non-enveloped viruses; and enveloped viruses. A revised hierarchy of susceptibility of pathogens to microbicides [7–10] spans the range of susceptibilities from most susceptible (enveloped viruses) to least susceptible (prions). This known hierarchy of susceptibility of pathogens to microbicides gives the public health community a starting point for IPAC countermeasures to be used for emerging pathogens, per the U.S. EPA [4].

2. The current WHO Priority List

The current WHO Priority disease list (**Box 1**) consists of viral diseases and Disease X, the latter being a placeholder that is always included in these lists. Disease X is used for the next unknown pathogen with the potential to cause a serious international epidemic. The viral families represented include *Arenaviridae* (Lassa fever virus); *Bunyaviridae* (Crimean-Congo hemorrhagic fever virus and Rift Valley fever virus); *Coronaviridae* (severe acute respiratory syndrome coronavirus 2 [SARS-CoV-2] causing COVID-19, Middle East respiratory syndrome coronavirus [MERS-CoV], and severe acute respiratory syndrome coronavirus [SARS-CoV]); *Filoviridae* (Ebola virus and Marburg virus]; *Flaviviridae* (Zika virus); and *Paramyxoviridae* (Nipah virus and henipaviruses).

Some of the characteristics of these viruses and their differences and commonalities are displayed in **Table 1**. Interestingly, these are each relatively

Virus	Family	Particle size	Lipid envelope	Genome[a] (segments)	Reservoir species	Reference(s)
Lassa virus	*Arenaviridae*	50–300 nm	Yes	±ssRNA(2)	Rodent	[11]
RVFV	*Bunyaviridae*	90–100 nm	Yes	−ssRNA(3)	Mosquito	[11]
CCHFV	*Bunyaviridae*	90–100 nm	Yes	−ssRNA(3)	Tick	[11]
MERS-CoV	*Coronaviridae*	90–130 nm	Yes	+ssRNA(1)	Bat	[12]
SARS-CoV	*Coronaviridae*	90–130 nm	Yes	+ssRNA(1)	Bat	[12]
SARS-CoV-2	*Coronaviridae*	90–130 nm	Yes	+ssRNA(1)	Bat[b]	[12]
Ebola virus	*Filoviridae*	80 × 14,000 nm	Yes	−ssRNA(1)	Bat	[11]
Marburg virus	*Filoviridae*	80 × 14,000 nm	Yes	−ssRNA(1)	Bat	[11]
Zika virus	*Flaviviridae*	50 nm	Yes	+ssRNA	Mosquito	[11]
Nipah virus	*Paramyxoviridae*	40–1900 nm	Yes	−ssRNA(1)	Bat	[13]

[a]*CCHFV, Crimean-Congo hemorrhagic fever virus; MERS-CoV, Middle East respiratory syndrome coronavirus; RVFV, Rift Valley fever virus; SARS-CoV, severe acute respiratory syndrome coronavirus; SARS-CoV-2, severe acute respiratory syndrome coronavirus 2; ±, ambisense; −, negative sense; +, positive sense; ss, single-stranded; segments (1) equates to a non-segmented genome.*
[b]*Suspected primary host [14].*

Table 1.
Characteristics of World Health Organization Priority List viruses.

large, lipid-enveloped viruses having single-stranded RNA genomes. Primary host infection of hemorrhagic viruses can be through insect vectors (arboviruses and flaviviruses), eating contaminated meat (filoviruses), consuming products in contact with bodily fluids of bats or pigs, such as blood, urine, nasal, respiratory droplets, and saliva (Nipah or henipaviruses), or exposure to contaminated rodent urine (Lassa virus). Once a human host is infected, the virus may be transmitted through contaminated bodily fluids and/or respiratory droplets. Non-hemorrhagic viruses such as SARS-CoV, SARS-CoV-2, and MERS-CoV are believed to be spread primarily by respiratory aerosols/droplets, although fomite transmission is also believed to play a role [10]. Case mortality rates vary, with SARS-CoV-2 having perhaps the lowest (2.1%), and Ebola Zaire virus among the highest (~90%). These viruses retain infectivity for hours to days after being deposited experimentally on non-porous surfaces [10].

The relatively high lethality of these viral diseases and the ability of the viruses to survive on surfaces [10] inform the need for effective hygiene interventions for interrupting the cycle of infection. Since these viruses have been placed on the WHO Priority List, one might assume that not much is known about virucidal efficacy of microbicides intended for surface hygiene, hand hygiene, and for rendering contaminated test samples safe for use in diagnostic testing for these viruses. In the remainder of this chapter, we review the information that is available on this topic, in order to address this assumption for the reader. The literature on SARS-CoV-2 virucidal efficacy is being updated continually, so the information presented in this chapter on SARS-CoV-2, specifically, should be considered a snapshot taken at the present point in time (i.e., September 2021).

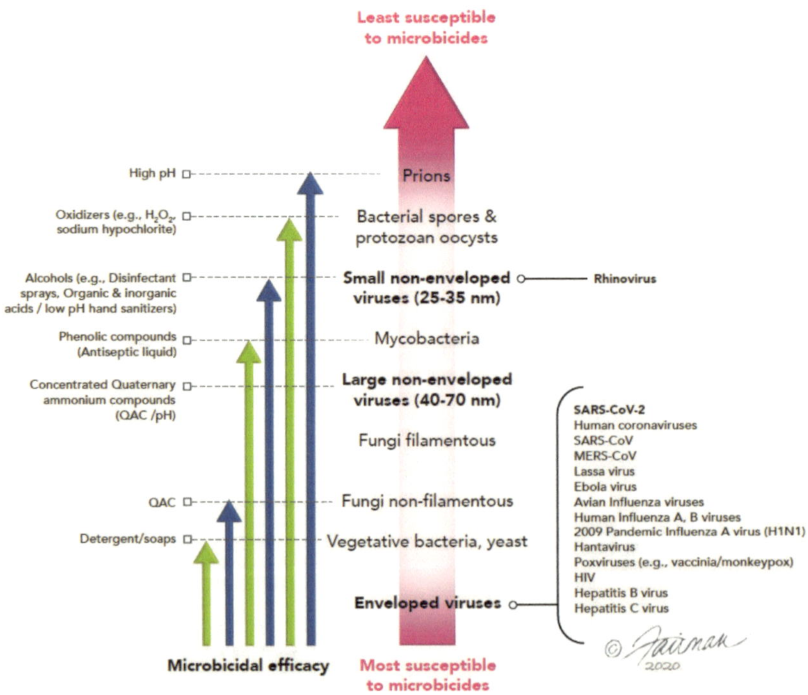

Figure 1.
Hierarchy of susceptibility of pathogens to microbicidal active ingredients. Certain formulated microbicides may include combinations of active ingredients, resulting in synergistic virucidal efficacy greater than that displayed by the individual active ingredients ([15] modified from Sattar [8]).

3. Predicted virucidal efficacy data for microbicides, including surface and hand hygiene agents, against the WHO Priority List viruses

The hierarchy of pathogen susceptibility to microbicides [5–10] (**Figure 1**) suggests that certain classes of microbicidal agents should display virucidal efficacy against lipid-enveloped viruses in general. For example, lipid-disrupting agents, such as alcohols, quaternary ammonium compounds (e.g., benzalkonium chloride), phenolics (e.g., para-chloro-meta-xylenol or PCMX), detergents (e.g., soap and Triton X-100), and organic acids (e.g., citric, lactic, and salicylic acids) would be expected to display similar virucidal efficacy for the WHO Priority List viruses, which are exclusively lipid-enveloped viruses. The same is true for protein-denaturing agents (alcohols, phenolics, oxidizers, and organic acids), and genome-degrading agents, such as alcohols and oxidizing agents. Of course, microbicides with virucidal efficacy against less susceptible pathogens, including mycobacteria, large and small non-enveloped viruses, and bacterial spores/protozoan oocysts, and prions, would certainly be expected to display virucidal efficacy against each of these WHO Priority List viruses. Having made these predictions, what do the empirical testing data tell us?

4. Empirical virucidal efficacy data for microbicides, including surface and hand hygiene agents, against the WHO Priority List viruses

In this section, we review the literature with regard to inactivation of WHO Priority List viruses by microbicides intended for decontamination of surfaces, for hand hygiene, for decontamination of liquids, and for test sample disinfection. Our discussion is limited to chemical microbicides, and specifically to the efficacy of these microbicides against the viruses mentioned in the WHO Priority List. The stated purpose of this review was to identify knowledge gaps for virucidal efficacy against the WHO Priority List viruses. As such, information pertaining to surrogate viruses from other families, or even unlisted viruses from the same families, is considered out of scope for this chapter. In addition, physical inactivation approaches (e.g., heating, ultraviolet radiation, and gamma irradiation), are not in scope for this chapter. A review of physical inactivation approaches for SARS-CoV-2 and other coronaviruses can be found in this book [16].

Inactivation studies evaluate pathogens dried onto a surface or within a suspension, but also may investigate efficacy for inactivating pathogens suspended in the air. Studies evaluating decontamination of surfaces involve the application of viruses, in the absence or presence of a soil load, onto carriers representing different prototypic environmental surfaces of interest (e.g., glass, stainless steel, plastic, etc.). Following drying of the applied virus onto the carrier for a set time period, a small quantity of the microbicide is added and left on for the specified contact (dwell) time. Residual virus is collected using an appropriate medium, and the titer post-treatment is compared to the initial untreated virus titer, with $\log_{10}$ reduction results accounting for any cytotoxicity of the test microbicide or neutralizing reagents used on the host cells used in the respective viral assays.

For suspension inactivation studies, depending on the test methodology chosen, virus is added to a liquid matrix, again in the absence or presence of a soil load. The microbicide is added at the evaluated test concentration and the solution is incubated at the appropriate temperature for the planned contact times. Again, the virus titers post-treatment are compared to the titer applied, with $\log_{10}$ reduction results accounting for any cytotoxicity of the test microbicide or neutralizing reagents used on the host cells used in the respective viral assays. Hand hygiene agents may be tested using suspension methodologies, or using specialized methods designed to recover virus directly from the skin. The hand hygiene agents are tested *in vitro*, or *in vivo* mimicking simulated-use (using *ex vivo* model), or under actual use-conditions in human volunteers. Efficacies of virucidal products intended for administration orally or nasally, and other types of therapeutic virucides, are not addressed in this review.

Because of the differences in testing methodologies used for evaluation of surface disinfection vs. decontamination of liquids or test samples, extrapolations of efficacy from one application to another should be made with caution. Differences in virucidal efficacy testing of microbicides (hand and surface hygiene agents) in liquid vs. on surfaces (inanimate or animate) have been identified, but these differences are typically relative, and may depend on the challenge virus and the microbicide being tested [17].

The virucidal efficacy literature for microbicides against Lassa virus is summarized in **Table 2**, and that for the bunyaviruses (Crimean-Congo hemorrhagic fever virus and Rift Valley fever virus) is summarized in **Table 3**. Information on virucidal efficacy for the coronaviruses (SARS-CoV-2, SARS-CoV, and MERS-CoV) is presented in **Table 4**, and virucidal efficacy for filoviruses (Ebola virus and Marburg virus) is shown in **Table 5**. **Table 6** presents virucidal efficacy data for the flavivirus (Zika virus), and the limited information on virucidal efficacy of microbicides against paramyxoviruses (Nipah virus and other henipaviruses) is summarized in **Table 7**.

Not all of the virucidal efficacy information from the reviewed articles is shown in **Tables 2–7**. Wherever possible, the virucidal efficacy data shown are from conditions leading to the highest $\log_{10}$ reduction level, or complete-inactivation of the challenge virus to the limit of detection of the infectivity assays used. No data from studies using exclusively nucleic acid assays have been included, as the nucleic

Virus/strain	Active ingredient	Product type	Contact time (min)[a]	Concentration in test	Efficacy ($\log_{10}$)[b]	Reference(s)
Surface hygiene						
			No literature found			
Hand hygiene						
			No literature found			
Suspension inactivation						
			No literature found			
Sample disinfection procedures						
Lassa Josiah	Acetic acid	Sample inactivant	15	3% (pH 2.5)	≥3	[18]
Lassa	Phenol/guanidine thiocyanate	Nucleic acid extractant	10	80% of neat	≥4.8	[19]
Lassa	β-Propiolactone	Sample inactivant	30 @ 37°C	0.2%	≥7	[20]
Lassa Josiah	Formalin	Cell fixative	20 days	Neat	Complete (cells)	[21]

[a]*Contact times at room temperature unless otherwise indicated.*
[b]*Inactivation matrix was virus stock (virus in culture medium), unless otherwise indicated.*

Table 2.
Efficacy of microbicides for inactivating the arenavirus Lassa virus.

Virus/ strain[a]	Active ingredient	Product type	Contact time (min)	Concentration in test	Efficacy (log_{10})[b]	Reference(s)
Surface hygiene						
			No literature found			
Hand hygiene						
			No literature found			
Suspension inactivation						
RVFV Menya/ Sheep/258	β-Propiolactone	Vaccine inactivant	240	3.5 mM	≥7	[22]
	Formalin	Vaccine inactivant	360	0.2%	>6	[22]
	Formalin	Vaccine inactivant				[23]
	Binary ethyleneamine	Vaccine inactivant				[23]
Sample disinfection procedures						
RVFV	Phenol/ guanidine thiocyanate	Nucleic acid extractant	10	80% of neat	≥6.8	[19]
RVFV	Formaldehyde	Cell fixative	1080	0.4%	≥7.0 (cells)	[24]
RVFV MP12	Formalin	Cell fixative	210 @ 4°C	Neat	Complete (cells)	[21]
CCHFV	FA Lysis Buffer	Sample inactivant	4	Undiluted	>4	[25]

[a]*CCHFV, Crimean-Congo hemorrhagic fever virus; RVFV, Rift Valley fever virus.*
[b]*Inactivation matrix was virus stock (virus in culture medium), unless otherwise indicated.*

Table 3.
Efficacy of microbicides for inactivating the bunyaviruses Rift Valley fever virus and Crimean-Congo hemorrhagic fever virus.

acid endpoints are not useful for measuring infectious virus unless integrated cell culture-qPCR based assays [58] are used. The individual reports in papers referenced in this chapter should be consulted for complete information, including concentration/response information, time/inactivation kinetics information, and microbicidal product names (which have not been included here).

4.1 Lassa virus

There have appeared in the literature only few reports of the empirical testing of microbicides for efficacy as virucides for the arenavirus (Lassa virus). The literature that has been identified has been summarized in **Table 2**. In addition, some descriptions of the utility of microbicides can be found in the secondary literature. For example [59], "LASV [Lassa virus] is susceptible to inactivation by most detergents and disinfectants. Sodium hypochlorite (0.5–1%), phenolic compounds, 3% acetic acid, lipid solvents and detergents (e.g., SDS), formaldehyde/paraformaldehyde, glutaraldehyde (2%), and beta-propiolactone disrupt virion integrity." The source provided for these claims was another secondary source [60]. No primary

Virus[a]	Active ingredient	Product type	Contact time (min)	Concentration in test	Efficacy (log_{10})	Reference(s)
Surface hygiene (glass or steel carriers)						
SARS-CoV-2	Ethanol, QAC (DBAS)	Disinfectant spray	1.75	50%, 0.08%	≥4.5	[15]
	QAC (DBAC)	Cleaner	2	0.09%	≥4.0	[15]
	QAC (DBAC)	Pre-impregnated wipes	1.75	0.19%	≥3.5	[15]
	Citric acid	Pre-impregnated wipes	0.5	2.4%	≥3.0	[15]
	Ethanol	Alcohol	1	70%	≥4.7	[26]
	Ethanol	Alcohol	1	70%	~5	[27]
	2-Propanol	Alcohol	1	70%	≥4.7	[26]
	2-Propanol	Alcohol	1	70%	~5	[27]
	Ethanol, 2-propanol	Alcohol	1	35%, 35%	~6	[27]
	H_2O_2	Microbicide	1	0.1%	≥4.5	[26]
	Sodium lauryl sulfate	Detergent	1	0.1%	≥4.6	[26]
SARS-CoV	Chloroxylenol (PCMX)	Antiseptic liquid	5	0.125%	≥6.0	[15]
	QAC (DBAC)	Dilutable cleaner	5	0.09%	≥4.8	[15]
	QAC (DBAC)	Cleaner	2	0.09%	≥3.8	[15]
	QAC (DBAC)	Pre-impregnated wipes	1.75	0.19%	≥5.8	[15]
	Citric acid	Pre-impregnated wipes	0.5	2.4%	≥3.0	[15]
MERS-CoV	Chloroxylenol (PCMX)	Antiseptic liquid	5	0.125%	≥5.0	[15]
Suspension inactivation						
SARS-CoV-2	Chloroxylenol (PCMX)	Antiseptic liquid	5	0.125%	≥6.0	[15]
	Chloroxylenol (PCMX)	Antiseptic liquid	1	0.125%	≥5.0	[15]
	Chloroxylenol (PCMX)	Antiseptic	5	0.05%	≥4.8	[28]
	Chlorhexidine	Cleaner	5	0.05%	≥4.8	[28]
	Trichloroisocyanuric acid	Microbicide	0.5	1000 mg/mL	≥4.8	[29]
	QAC (DBAC)	Surface cleanser	5	0.077%	≥4.1	[15]
	QAC (BKC)	Cleaner	5	0.45%	≥4.5	[15]
	QAC (BKC)	Antiseptic	5	0.1%	≥4.8	[28]
	QAC (DNB)	Cleaner	0.5	283 mg/mL	≥4.9	[29]

Virus[a]	Active ingredient	Product type	Contact time (min)	Concentration in test	Efficacy (log_{10})	Reference(s)
	QAC (DNC)	Cleaner	0.5	283 mg/mL	≥4.9	[29]
	Lactic acid	Surface cleanser	5	1.9%	≥5.5	[15]
	Sodium hypochlorite	Dilutable cleaner	0.5	0.14%	≥5.1	[15]
	Sodium hypochlorite	Bathroom cleaner	5	0.32%	≥5.1	[15]
	Sodium hypochlorite	Household bleach	5	1:49	≥4.8	[28]
	Sodium hypochlorite	Household bleach	1	9%	≥3.3	[30]
	Hydrochloric acid	Toilet bowl cleaner	0.5	0.25%	≥4.1	[15]
	Ethanol	Disinfectant spray	5	48%	≥4.1	[15]
	Ethanol	**Alcohol**	**5**	**63%**	**≥4.8**	**[28]**
	Ethanol	**Alcohol**	**0.5**	**30%**	**≥5.9**	**[31]**
	Ethanol	**Alcohol**	**0.5**	**40%**	**≥4.8**	**[29]**
	Ethanol	**Alcohol**	**5**	**68%**	**≥2.00**	**[30]**
	2-Propanol	**Alcohol**	**0.5**	**30%**	**≥5.9**	**[31]**
	Copper-iodine	PPE disinfectant	30	90%	≥3.5	[32]
	Povidone-iodine	Antiseptic	5	7.5%	≥4.8	[28]
	Povidone-iodine	Antiseptic	0.5	10%	≥4.0	[33]
	Formaldehyde	**Microbicide**	**1**	**10%**	**≥1.3**	**[30]**
	Formaldehyde	**Microbicide**	**15**	**2%**	**≥4.8**	**[34]**
SARS-CoV	**2-Propanol**	**Alcohol**	**0.5**	**80%**	**≥3.3**	**[35]**
	2-Propanol	**Alcohol**	**0.5**	**56%**	**≥3.3**	**[35]**
	Ethanol, 2-biphenylol	Microbicide	0.5	50%, 0.16%	≥5.0	[35]
	QAC (BKC), laurylamine	Microbicide	30	0.5%	≥6.1	[36]
	QAC (BKC), glutaraldehyde	Microbicide	30	0.5%	≥3.8	[36]
	Magnesium monoperphthalate	**Microbicide**	**30**	**0.5%**	**≥4.5**	**[36]**
	Glutaraldehyde (ethylendioxy) dimethanol	Instrument disinfectant	15	2%	≥3.3	[36]
	Povidone-iodine	**Antiseptic**	**1**	**1%**	**4.1**	**[37]**
Hand hygiene agents						
SARS-CoV-2	Chloroxylenol (PCMX)	Bar soap	0.5	0.014%	≥4.1	[15]
	Chloroxylenol (PCMX)	Antiseptic liquid	5	0.021%	≥4.7	[15]

Virus[a]	Active ingredient	Product type	Contact time (min)	Concentration in test	Efficacy (log_{10})	Reference(s)
	Chlorhexidine gluconate	Disinfectant	1	1.0%	3.2	[38]
	Soap	Liquid hand soap	1	90%	≥2.0	[30]
	Soap	Bar soap	0.33	8%	≥3.1	[27]
	Ethanol	Hand sanitizer gel	1	53%	≥4.2	[15]
	Ethanol	Hand sanitizer gel	1	53%	≥4.2	[15]
	Ethanol	Hand sanitizer	1	63%	≥2.5	[30]
	Ethanol	Hand sanitizer gel	0.5	70%	≥3.2	[39]
	Ethanol	Hand sanitizer foam	0.5	70%	≥3.2	[39]
	Ethanol	Hand sanitizer	0.17	65%	≥4.0	[27]
	Ethanol	**Alcohol**	**0.08**	**40%**	**≥4.2**	**[38]**
	2-Propanol	**Alcohol**	**0.08**	**70%**	**≥4.2**	**[38]**
	Salicyclic acid	Liquid gel handwash	0.5	0.025%	≥3.6	[15]
	QAC (BKC)	Foaming handwash	1	0.025%	≥3.4	[15]
	QAC (BKC)	Disinfectant	1	0.2%	3.2	[27]
	Salicyclic acid	Foaming handwash	0.5	0.023%	≥5.0	[15]
	Citric acid, lactic acid	Hand sanitizer gel	0.5	1.5%, 0.41%	≥4.7	[15]
	Povidone-iodine	Skin cleanser	0.5	7.5%	≥4.0	[33]
	Ethanol, H_2O_2	WHO formulation I hand rub (original)	1	72%, 0.1%	≥2.2	[30]
	Ethanol, H_2O_2	WHO formulation I hand rub (original)	0.5	64%, 0.1%	≥3.8	[31]
	Ethanol, H_2O_2	WHO formulation I hand rub (modified)	0.5	64%, 0.1%	≥5.9	[31]
	2-Propanol, H_2O_2	WHO formulation II hand rub (original)	0.5	60%, 0.1%	≥3.8	[31]
	2-Propanol, H_2O_2	WHO formulation II hand rub (modified)	0.5	60%, 0.1%	≥5.9	[31]

Virus[a]	Active ingredient	Product type	Contact time (min)	Concentration in test	Efficacy (log_{10})	Reference(s)
SARS-CoV	Ethanol, H_2O_2	WHO formulation I hand rub (original)	0.5	32%, 0.05%	≥5	[40]
	2-Propanol, H_2O_2	WHO formulation II hand rub (original)	0.5	24%, 0.04%	≥5	[40]
	2-Propanol, 1-propanol	Hand rub	0.5	36%, 24%	≥2.8	[35]
	2-Propanol, 1-propanol	Hand rub	0.5	36%, 24%	≥4.3	[35]
	Ethanol	Hand rub	0.5	64%	≥4.3	[35]
	Ethanol	Hand rub	0.5	68%	≥5.5	[35]
	Ethanol	Hand rub	0.5	76%	≥5.5	[35]
MERS-CoV	Ethanol, H_2O_2	WHO formulation I hand rub (original)	0.5	32%, 0.05%	≥5	[40]
	2-Propanol, H_2O_2	WHO formulation II hand rub (original)	0.5	32%, 0.05%	≥5	[40]
	Povidone-iodine	Surgical scrub	0.25	7.5%	4.6	[41]
	Povidone-iodine	Skin cleanser	0.25	4%	5.0	[41]
	Povidone-iodine	Scrub	1	1%	≥6.1	[41]
	Povidone-iodine	Scrub	1	0.25%	≥6.1	[41]
Sample disinfection procedures						
SARS-CoV-2	Sodium dodecyl sulfate	Detergent	30	0.5%	≥4	[42]
	Sodium dodecyl sulfate	Detergent	30	10%	5.7	[34]
	Triton X-100	Detergent	30	0.5%	≥4	[42]
	Triton X-100	Detergent	30	10%	≥4.9	[34]
	NP-40	Detergent	30	0.5%	≥4	[42]
	NP-40	Detergent	30	10%	≥6.5	[34]
	Methanol	Tissue fixative	30	100%	≥6.0	[42]
	Methanol	Cell fixative	15	100%	≥6.7	[34]
	p-Formaldehyde	Tissue fixative	30	4%	≥6.0	[42]
	Formaldehyde	Cell fixative	60	10%	6	[43]
	Formaldehyde	Cell fixative	60	4%	≥7.5	[33]
	Phenol/guanidine thiocyanate	Nucleic acid extractant	5	80%	≥4	[42]
	Phenol/guanidine thiocyanate	Nucleic acid extractant	5	80%	≥4	[42]

Virus[a]	Active ingredient	Product type	Contact time (min)	Concentration in test	Efficacy (log_{10})	Reference(s)
	Phenol/guanidine thiocyanate	Nucleic acid extractant	10	0.5%	6	[43]
	Beta-propiolactone	Inactivant for vaccines	960	0.05%	6	[43]
	Polyhexamethylene biguanide	Cell lysis buffer	30	2%	1.6	[34]
SARS-CoV	Methanol	Tissue fixative	30	100%	≥6.0	[37]
	Methanol	Cell fixative	30	100%	≥6.0	[37]
	Acetone	Cell fixative	30	100%	≥6.0	[37]
	p-Formaldehyde	Tissue fixative	5	3.5%	≥3.7	[37]
	Formaldehyde	Tissue fixative	2	0.7%	≥3.0	[35]
	Glutaraldehyde	Tissue fixative	15	2.5%	≥4.4	[37]
MERS-CoV	Phenol/guanidine thiocyanate	Nucleic acid extractant	10	80%	≥6.1	[18]

[a]BKC, benzalkonium chloride; DBAC, dimethyl benzyl ammonium chloride; DBAS, dimethyl benzyl ammonium saccharinate; DNB, di-N-decyl dimethyl ammonium bromide; DNC, di-N-decyl dimethyl ammonium chloride; H_2O_2, hydrogen peroxide; MERS-CoV, Middle East respiratory syndrome coronavirus; ND, not determined; PBS, phosphate buffered saline; SARS-CoV, severe acute respiratory syndrome coronavirus; SARS-CoV-2, severe acute respiratory syndrome coronavirus 2; WHO, World Health Organization. Entries in blue font indicate formulations with microbicidal active ingredients.

Table 4.
Efficacy of microbicides for inactivating the coronaviruses SARS-CoV-2, SARS-CoV, and MERS-CoV.

literature source was provided for these claims, and it should be noted that important information such as contact times, temperatures, inactivation matrices, or methodologies was not provided in these secondary sources [59, 60].

No primary literature (peer-reviewed) for virucidal efficacy of Lassa virus by microbicides on surfaces or in suspensions, or for efficacy of hand hygiene agents was identified during this literatures search. Characterization of the efficacy of microbicides for these purposes is required to resolve this knowledge gap. The few reports found related to agents intended for rendering laboratory samples safe for use in diagnostic assays [18–21].

4.2 Crimean-Congo hemorrhagic fever virus and Rift Valley fever virus

There are few reports of the empirical testing of microbicides for efficacy as virucides for the bunyaviruses [Crimean-Congo hemorrhagic fever virus (CCHFV) and Rift Valley fever virus (RVFV)]. The literature that has been identified has been summarized in **Table 3**. In addition, some descriptions of disinfectant utility can be found in the secondary literature. For example, "CCHFV can be inactivated by many disinfectants including 1% hypochlorite, 70% alcohol, hydrogen peroxide, peracetic acid, iodophors, glutaraldehyde, and formalin" [61]. No primary literature source was provided for these claims, and it should be noted that important information such as contact times, temperatures, inactivation matrices, or methodologies was not provided in this brief description [61]. Similar information is provided in the review by Bartoli et al. [62]. In that review, which has an emphasis on laboratory safety, attribution to the primary literature for CCHFV is provided for

Virus/ variant[a]	Active ingredients	Product type	Contact time (min)	Concentration in test	Efficacy (log_{10})[b]	Reference(s)
Surface hygiene (steel or aluminum carriers)						
Ebola Makona	Sodium hypochlorite	Microbicide	5	0.5%	≥6.6	[44]
	Sodium hypochlorite	Microbicide	5	0.5%	≥6.8	[45]
	Sodium hypochlorite	Microbicide	15	0.5%	≥2.0	[46]
	Sodium hypochlorite	Microbicide	15	0.5%	<1 (blood)	[46]
	Sodium hypochlorite	Microbicide	5	0.5%	≥5.1	[47]
	Sodium hypochlorite	Pre-impregnated wipe	0.08	1%	6.3	[48]
	Ethanol	Alcohol	5	67%	≥7.3	[44]
	Ethanol	Alcohol	2.5	70%	≥6.8	[45]
	Ethanol	Alcohol	5	70%	≥6.9	[47]
	Ethanol	Disinfectant spray	5	58%	≥4.5	[47]
	Ethanol	Pre-impregnated wipe	0.08	66.5%	6.6	[48]
	Ethanol	Alcohol	2	70%	1.7	[46]
	Ethanol	Alcohol	2	70%	<1 (blood)	[46]
	Peracetic acid	Microbicide	5	5%	≥1.0	[46]
	Peracetic acid	Microbicide	5	5%	≥2.0 (blood)	[46]
	Chloroxylenol (PCMX)	Microbicide	5	0.48%	≥5.1	[47]
	H_2O_2	Pre-impregnated wipe	1	2.5%	6.4	[48]
	H_2O_2, peroxyacetic acid	Microbicide	5	Undiluted	2.6	[46]
	H_2O_2, peroxyacetic acid	Microbicide	5	Undiluted	<1 (blood)	[46]
	QAC	Microbicide	10	1.5%	<1	[46]
	QAC	Pre-impregnated wipe	1	As supplied	6.6	[48]
	QAC	Pre-impregnated wipe	0.08	5%	6.0	[48]
Ebola Mayinga	Sodium hypochlorite	Microbicide	5	0.5%	≥6.6	[45]
	Ethanol	Alcohol	1	70%	≥6.6	[45]
Ebola Kikwit	Sodium hypochlorite	Microbicide	5	0.5%	≥6.5	[45]
	Ethanol	Alcohol	1	70%	≥6.5	[45]
Ebola Yambuku-Ecran	Sodium hypochlorite	Microbicide	10	0.75%	≥6.5	[49]

Virus/ variant[a]	Active ingredients	Product type	Contact time (min)	Concentration in test	Efficacy (log_{10})[b]	Reference(s)
	Alcohol formulation	Microbicide	10	50%	5.3	[42]
	QAC, alcohol	Microbicide	10	1.5%	2.5	[42]
	QAC, alkylamine	Microbicide	10	2.5%	4.2	[42]
Suspension inactivation						
Ebola Makona	Chloroxylenol (PCMX)	Antiseptic liquid	1	0.48%	≥4.8	[50]
Ebola Zaire	Povidone-iodine	Microbicide	0.25	1:10+	≥5.5	[51]
Hand hygiene agents						
Ebola Makona	Salicylic acid, citric acid	Liquid hand wash	0.5	1:4	4.8	[52]
Ebola Zaire	Povidone-iodine	Skin cleanser	0.5	1:10	≥4.5	[51]
	Povidone-iodine	Surgical scrub	0.25	1:10	≥5.5	[51]
	Povidone-iodine, alcohol	Skin cleanser	0.25	Undiluted	≥5.7	[51]
Ebola Mayinga	Ethanol, H_2O_2	WHO formulation I hand rub (original)	0.5	32%, 0.05%	≥5	[40]
	2-Propanol, H_2O_2	WHO formulation II hand rub (original)	0.5	24%, 0.04%	≥5	[40]
Sample disinfection procedures						
Ebola	Triton X-100	Detergent	60	0.1%	4	[53]
Ebola Makona	Triton X-100	Detergent	60	0.1%	≥3 (FBS)	[54]
	Phenol/guanidine thiocyanate	Nucleic acid extractant	10	80% of neat	≥5.5	[19]
	Sodium dodecyl sulfate	Detergent	60	0.1%	≥3 (FBS)	[54]
	Sodium dodecyl sulfate	Detergent	60	0.1%	~1 (blood)	[54]
Ebola Sudan	Phenol/guanidine thiocyanate	Nucleic acid extractant	10	80% of neat	≥4.5	[19]
Ebola Mayinga	Acetic acid	Sample inactivant	15	3% (pH 2.5)	≥3 (blood)	[18]
Marburg Ci67	Phenol/guanidine thiocyanate	Nucleic acid extractant	10	80% of neat	≥6.1	[19]
Marburg Musokee	Acetic acid	Sample inactivant	15	3% (pH 2.5)	≥3	[18]

[a]*FBS, fetal bovine serum; H_2O_2, hydrogen peroxide; QAC, quaternary ammonium compound; WHO, World Health Organization. Entries in blue font indicate formulations with microbicidal active ingredients.*
[b]*Inactivation matrix was virus stock (virus in culture medium), unless otherwise indicated.*

Table 5.
Efficacy of microbicides for inactivating the filoviruses Ebola and Marburg viruses.

one of the eight references supporting the disinfectant efficacy section. The remaining references are either secondary literature or are related to the filovirus Ebola virus, not to CCHFV. Thus, the same disinfectant efficacy data, for which

Virus/ strain	Active ingredient	Product type	Contact time (min)	Concentration in test	Efficacy (log_{10})	Reference(s)
Surface hygiene (glass or plastic carriers)						
Zika virus PRVABC59	2-Propanol	Alcohol	0.25	70%	≥5.1	[55]
					≥5.6 (blood)	[55]
	QAC[a]/2-propanol	Microbicide	0.25	Undiluted	≥3.5	[55]
					≥3.4 (blood)	[55]
	Peracetic acid	Microbicide	5	1000 ppm	≥4.9	[55]
					1.4 (blood)	[55]
	Chlorine	Microbicide	5	500 ppm	≥4.1	[55]
					0.1 (blood)	[55]
Zika virus MR 766	Sodium hypochlorite	Microbicide	1	1%	>3	[56]
	Ethanol	Commercial alcohol	1	70%	>3	[56]
	2 Propanol	Commercial alcohol	1	70%	>3	[56]
	Paraformaldehyde	Microbicide	1	2%	>3	[56]
	Glutaraldehyde	Tissue fixative	1	2%	>3	[56]
Suspension inactivation						
Zika virus MR 766	Sodium hypochlorite	Microbicide	1	0.70%	>6	[56]
	Ethanol	Microbicide	1	49%	>6	[56]
	2-Propanol	Microbicide	1	49%	>6	[56]
	Paraformaldehyde	Microbicide	1	1.4%	>6	[56]
	Glutaraldehyde	Tissue fixative	1	1.4%	>6	[56]
Hand hygiene agents						
Zika virus MP 1751	Ethanol, H_2O_2	WHO formulation I hand rub (original)	0.5	32%, 0.05%	≥5	[40]
	2-Propanol, H_2O_2	WHO formulation II hand rub (original)	0.5	24%, 0.05%	≥5	[40]
Sample disinfection procedures						
Zika virus PRVABC59	β-Propiolactone	Microbicide	180	3%	>7	[57]
	Ethanol	Alcohol	5	35%	>7	[57]
	Ethanol	Alcohol	2	58%	>7	[57]
	QAC[a]	Microbicide	2	2.5%	>7	[57]
	QAC[a]	Microbicide	1	4.2%	>7	[57]
	QAC[a]	Microbicide	2	50%	>7	[57]

[a]QAC, quaternary ammonium compound: n-alkyl dimethyl benzyl ammonium chloride, n-alkyl ethyl benzyl ammonium chloride; H_2O_2, hydrogen peroxide; WHO, World Health Organization. Entries in blue font indicate formulations with microbicidal active ingredients.

Table 6.
Efficacy of microbicides for inactivating the flavivirus Zika virus.

Virus/ strain[a]	Active ingredient	Product type	Contact time (min)	Concentration in test	Efficacy (log_{10})	Reference(s)
Surface hygiene						
			No literature found			
Suspension inactivation						
			No literature found			
Hand hygiene agents						
			No literature found			
			Sample disinfection procedures			
Nipah	Phenol/guanidine thiocyanate	Sample inactivant	10	80% of neat	≥6.0	[19]

Table 7.
Efficacy of microbicides for inactivating the paramyxoviruses Nipah virus and other henipaviruses.

primary supporting data do not appear to be available, have appeared in numerous secondary sources and review articles on RVFV or CCHFV.

No primary reports describing efficacy of microbicides as surface or hand hygiene agents, or for inactivating these viruses in suspensions were identified during the literature search (**Table 3**). This represents a significant knowledge gap with respect to IPAC for these viruses. The available inactivation efficacy data relate to vaccine virus inactivation [22, 23] and sample disinfection reagents/cell fixatives [19, 21, 24, 25] for RVFV or CCHFV. The few microbicides that have been evaluated are solvents or detergents with expected efficacy for inactivating an enveloped virus, such as a bunyavirus.

4.3 SARS-CoV-2, SARS-CoV, and MERS-CoV

In the case of SARS-CoV-2, an extensive literature for virucidal efficacy of microbicides has been developed over the past year and a half. To a lesser extent, literature for original SARS-CoV and for MERS-CoV was identified. Data on the inactivation of these beta-coronaviruses by microbicides are summarized in **Table 4**. The information displayed in **Table 4** considers microbicides intended for disinfection of HITES [15, 26, 27], inactivation in liquid suspension [15, 28–37], and microbicides intended for hand hygiene [15, 27, 30, 31, 33, 35, 38–41, 63] and for laboratory sample decontamination [19, 34, 35, 37, 42, 43]. Additional reports on disinfection of laboratory samples which did not report results in terms of log_{10} reduction in titer include the following [64, 65]. The inactivation literature for SARS-CoV-2 and other coronaviruses has been reviewed extensively [66–75]. Readers interested in the virucidal efficacy of these microbicides for coronaviruses under different testing conditions, carrier types, contact times, temperatures, and the presence or absence of a challenge soil load are advised to examine these review papers, as well as the primary literature sources indicated in **Table 4**. It was not possible to display all useful information from these sources within one summary table, so **Table 4** should be used as a guide for pursuing additional detail for the listed microbicides and applications.

The types of microbicides that display virucidal efficacy for SARS-CoV-2, SARS-CoV, and MERS-CoV-2 are those expected to be lipid-disrupting agents (e.g., solvents, alcohols, detergents, phenolics, and quaternary ammonium compounds) and broad-spectrum microbicides (oxidizing agents, and organic and inorganic acids and bases). Inactivation conditions leading to complete inactivation to the limit of detection of the infectivity assays have been described in **Table 4**, enabling researchers and healthcare workers to implement cleaning regimens with the greatest chances of limiting onward transmission of the virus through contaminated fomites, solutions, hands, and diagnostic samples. The primary knowledge gap identified during this literature review is around the efficacy of plain soap and water inactivation of the beta-coronaviruses. This gap has been discussed previously [76].

4.4 Ebola virus and Marburg virus

Ebola virus and Marburg virus are members of the *Filoviridae* family. These are enveloped viruses which cause relatively lethal hemorrhagic fevers in humans. Most of the available literature on inactivation of Ebola virus variants by microbicides has been generated in carrier studies [44–49]. Very little data for inactivation of Ebola virus in suspension studies was identified during the literature search [50, 51]. Few reports of the efficacy of hand hygiene agents for inactivating Ebola virus were found [40, 51, 52], while efficacy of laboratory sample decontamination agents has been reported both for Ebola virus variants [18, 19, 53, 54] and Marburg virus strains [18, 19]. The data from these reports have been summarized in **Table 5**. Fortunately, a variety of Ebola variants have been used as challenge viruses, and at least two strains of Marburg virus have been evaluated. Where side-by-side comparisons of efficacy between variants has been evaluated [45], any differences in virucidal efficacy identified have been relative; that is, differences have been in degree of inactivation (i.e., $\log_{10}$ reduction in titer) only.

Knowledge gaps for Ebola virus inactivation include evaluation of the efficacy of plain soap and water hand washing. In the case of Marburg virus, little virucidal-efficacy data of microbicides (surface and hand hygiene agents) have been generated. This knowledge gap is, therefore, relatively profound. The secondary literature [77] suggests that "Ebola viruses and Marburg viruses are both reported to be susceptible to sodium hypochlorite, glutaraldehyde, β-propiolactone, 3% acetic acid (pH 2.5), formaldehyde, and paraformaldehyde. Recommended dilutions of sodium hypochlorite may vary with the use. Calcium hypochlorite, peracetic acid, methyl alcohol, ether, sodium deoxycholate, and some other agents have also been tested against Ebola viruses, and found to be effective." The only source provided in support of the above was Mitchell and McCormick [18]. As is apparent, much of the current knowledge in such secondary sources [77, 78] pertains to inactivating agents for rendering laboratory samples safe for use. It should be noted that for most of the listed microbicides, important information such as microbicide concentration, contact time, temperature, inactivation matrix, or study methodology was not provided in these secondary sources.

4.5 Zika virus

Zika virus is a member of the *Flaviviridae* family of enveloped viruses, which includes such common pathogens as hepatitis C virus, West Nile virus, hog cholera virus, and bovine viral diarrhea virus. Data on the inactivation of Zika virus by microbicides have been summarized in **Table 6**. The information displayed in **Table 6** considers microbicides intended for surface disinfection [55, 56], inactivation in liquid suspension [56], and microbicides intended for hand hygiene [40], and for laboratory sample decontamination [57]. While the totality of the data is relatively minimal, a variety of lipid-disrupting agents have been evaluated and found effective. The oxidizing agents (chlorine, sodium hypochlorite, and hydrogen peroxide) also proved effective, as expected per the hierarchy of susceptibility to microbicides (**Figure 1**). Note that the peracetic acid- and chlorine-containing microbicides displayed limited efficacy when the virus was dried on carriers within a blood matrix (**Table 6**). Since Zika virus is transmitted primarily through insect vectors and fomite (indirect) transmission plays a lesser role, the surface hygiene, suspension inactivation, and hand hygiene efficacy data are mainly relevant to IPAC under health-care and laboratory settings (i.e., handling clinical samples containing bodily fluids for analysis). Relevance for the public-at-large is perhaps lesser, compared with the other viruses discussed within this chapter.

4.6 Nipah virus and other henipaviruses

Very little information on the virucidal efficacy of microbicides for Nipah virus or other henipaviruses was identified during this literature search. Claims as to utility of certain microbicides for these paramyxoviruses include the following: "Paramyxoviruses are susceptible to common soaps and disinfectants; lipid solvents (alcohol and ether) and sodium hypochlorite solutions were used effectively in outbreaks for cleaning and disinfection" [79]. This sort of information, without supporting primary literature, is only marginally useful. Important information, including microbicide concentration, contact time, matrix and methodology used to determine virucidal efficacy, are missing from this brief statement. It is clear from **Table 7** that considerable knowledge gaps exist for virucidal efficacy of microbicides for these Priority List paramyxoviruses.

5. Discussion

In the case of IPAC, it is common for microbicidal actives to be formulated into products intended for surface or hand hygiene. These products are used to interrupt the cycle of infection involving the indirect transfer of virus from contaminated fomites to the hand and then to mucous membranes of a susceptible individual. There is also the possibility of re-aerosolization of virus from a contaminated fomite [80–84], potentially leading to direct airborne transmission to mucous membranes of a susceptible person. As mentioned in the preceding sections, these routes of infection may be less important for those viruses that are primarily transmitted through insect vectors (e.g., Zika virus). Microbicides are typically used for all of the WHO Priority List viruses *as is* for disinfection of laboratory samples to render them safe for handling.

The stated purpose of this review was to identify gaps in the current state of the science regarding the virucidal efficacy of microbicides (including surface and hand hygiene agents) for viruses causing the current WHO Priority List diseases. The viruses that cause Priority List diseases are also mentioned in lists of pathogens of concern issued by other health agencies globally. For instance, Lassa virus, Rift Valley fever virus, Crimean-Congo hemorrhagic fever virus, Ebola virus, and Marburg virus are also mentioned in the National Institute of Allergy and Infectious Diseases (NIAID) Emerging Infectious Diseases/Pathogens priority A list [85]. The NIAID list was issued in 2018 and, therefore, did not include SARS-CoV-2. SARS-CoV-2 is certainly now a priority virus for NIAID [86]. A discussion of emerging and re-emerging viruses can be found in Morens and Fauci [87]. Listed among other emerging viruses in that review are SARS-CoV, MERS-CoV, SARS-CoV-2, Zika virus, Rift Valley fever virus; Nipah virus, Hendra virus, Ebola virus, and Marburg virus. Additional viruses not mentioned in the WHO Priority List include additional bunyaviruses, influenza virus strains, enteroviruses and poxviruses [87]. A recent review of emerging and re-emerging viral infections by Schwartz [88] also mentions, among other viruses, Lassa virus, Ebola virus, Marburg virus, Zika virus, SARS-CoV-2, MERS-CoV, and SARS-CoV, and Rift Valley fever virus. Knowledge gaps outlined in that review did not include gaps in information on disinfection/ surface hygiene and hand hygiene. The WHO also maintains what is referred to as an "R&D Blueprint" and an "R&D Roadmap" to provide guidance on appropriate responses to Priority List disease outbreaks and to develop ways to improve global responses to future epidemics [89]. This was last updated in 2017 and, therefore, is not as current as the WHO Priority List. The R&D Blueprint also is more a description of the types of knowledge gaps for epidemic preparedness (vaccine testing, diagnostic technologies, therapeutic interventions, vector control) than a list of viruses of concern [89].

It was assumed at the time of undertaking this literature review that, by definition, information would be minimal for at least some of the Priority List viruses (**Table 1**), and this indeed turned out to be the case. Although it is clear that knowledge for one member of a given virus family should be informative for other members of the same virus family, the purpose of this review was to identify knowledge gaps for the specific viruses of concern, not to review inactivation information for surrogate viruses from the same or other viruses from the families (**Table 1**). Such an exercise, while of value for IPAC of these specific viruses, was considered to be well beyond the scope of this chapter. Readers interested in identifying microbicides with efficacy for inactivating any of the Priority List viruses are encouraged to review the literature cited in this chapter, to consider the predictions of virucidal efficacy discussed in Section 3 of this chapter, and to search and review the literature for inactivation of other members of the virus family of interest.

It can be safely said that, following these steps, one may arrive at a list of microbicides and conditions (temperature, microbicide concentration, contact time, testing matrix, etc.) that should adequately inactivate each of the Priority List viruses. As an example, there are extremely limited data for the paramyxoviruses Nipah virus and other henipaviruses. There are, however, a variety of other paramyxoviruses for which inactivation data are available, and the lipid-disrupting agents and broad-spectrum microbicides effective against the less lethal paramyxoviruses (e.g., respiratory syncytial virus, parainfluenza virus type 3) should be equally effective against the Priority List paramyxoviruses.

It is clear that during the ongoing SARS-CoV-2 pandemic, the majority of the resources of the public health community were applied to research into one or more of the many different aspects of SARS-CoV-2 for IPAC. In fact, many laboratories have been conducting research exclusively on SARS-CoV-2 during the ongoing pandemic. Because of this, literature on all aspects of the virus and the disease, COVID-19, has appeared on a relatively continuous basis. The relatively great amount of empirical data collected to date on the virucidal efficacy of microbicides for SARS-CoV-2, SARS-CoV, and MERS-CoV (**Table 4**) reflects this emphasis. Of course, during a pandemic impacting ~435 million confirmed cases globally and ~5.9 million global deaths as of February 28, 2022 [90], this universal focus on the virus and the disease was, and remains, appropriate, particularly with the emergence of Delta, Omicron, and other variants [91, 92].

It is also clear from this review of the literature on the virucidal efficacy of microbicides for the WHO Priority List viruses that relatively limited information is available on some viruses, especially the paramyxoviruses Nipah virus and related henipaviruses and the bunyaviruses CCHFV and RVFV. Rift Valley fever virus and CCHFV are infectious agents considered as bioterrorism threats, due in part to the paucity of knowledge on measures for mitigating the transmission of the viruses and severity of the associated diseases [93, 94]. Reviews of focus areas and knowledge gaps for CCHFV [93–95] mention tick (vector) surveillance and vector control agents, but does not discuss knowledge gaps around surface disinfection or hand hygiene. For the arboviruses (Rift Valley fever virus, Crimean-Congo hemorrhagic fever virus, Zika virus), the possibility of contamination of high-touch environmental surfaces with patient blood spills and other patient excretions/secretions needs to be considered and transmission risk mitigated through application of effective microbicides. Further research into this topic is, therefore, required. For surface virucidal studies, the impact of the matrix in which the challenge virus is suspended at time of drying on the carrier should always be evaluated. As shown in the Zika surface inactivation studies (**Table 6**), virus deposited in a blood matrix does not appear to be effectively inactivated by the microbicides peracetic acid and chlorine, compared to inactivation of virus dried in the absence of the blood load [55].

It is to be expected that, as the current pandemic wanes, research into the more lethal, albeit less common, viral diseases mentioned in this chapter will be encouraged and undertaken at the BSL-3 and BSL-4 laboratories capable of safely handling these viruses. For instance, further studies need to be carried out on the virucidal efficacy of commonly used microbicides (surface and hand hygiene agents) for Lassa virus and Nipah virus in surface and suspension inactivation studies. This information will provide additional confirmation of the expectation that microbicides capable of inactivating enveloped viruses, in general, should be effective for these Priority List viruses. Until such data are generated, the IPAC community will continue to be able to leverage virucidal efficacy data for other enveloped and non-enveloped viruses per the Emerging Viral Pathogen Guidance for Antimicrobial Pesticides from the U.S. EPA [4, 5] and the European tiered approach for virucidal efficacy testing [96].

6. Conclusions

In this chapter, we have reviewed the current state of the science regarding the virucidal efficacy of microbicides for viruses causing the current WHO Priority List diseases. By definition, information might be expected to be minimal for at least some of these viruses, hence the need for encouraging additional research. Not surprisingly, the efficacy of microbicides for inactivation of certain of the lethal (BSL-4) viruses, especially the paramyxoviruses Nipah virus and related henipaviruses and the bunyaviruses CCHFV and RVFV, was found to be poorly characterized. The need for further research into the virucidal efficacy of microbicides for the arenavirus (Lassa virus) and the filovirus (Marburg virus) is also indicated by the relative paucity of empirical data identified during the review. For the beta-coronaviruses (SARS-CoV, SARS-CoV-2, and MERS-CoV), the filovirus (Ebola virus), and the flavivirus (Zika virus), the available knowledge base for virucidal efficacy of microbicides appears to be adequate for verifying the predicted efficacy based on the hierarchy of virus susceptibility to microbicides.

It is hoped that this discussion will provide assurance to the IPAC community of the empirically determined virucidal efficacy of targeted hygiene agents against SARS-CoV-2 for use during the current SARS-CoV-2/COVID-19 pandemic. SARS-CoV-2 is evolving continuously, and the emerging mutational variants are being monitored for impact on previously vaccinated and non-vaccinated individuals. The microbicides displaying virucidal efficacy against SARS-CoV-2, MERS-CoV, and SARS-CoV should display equivalent efficacy against emerging mutational variants [97], including the Delta, Omicron, and other variants. Current Variants of Interest (VOI) may become Variants of Concern (VOC) in the future, and the appropriate CDC/WHO websites [91, 92] should be consulted to keep up-to-date regarding the mutational variants of SARS-CoV-2. The information presented in this chapter also should be useful for the IPAC community as it considers non-pharmaceutical interventions for the other Priority List diseases in addition to SARS-CoV-2.

Acknowledgements

The authors thank Drs. Chris Jones and Mark Ripley, Reckitt Benckiser R&D, for their critical review of the manuscript.

Conflict of interest

Drs. Julie McKinney and M. Khalid Ijaz are engaged in R&D at Reckitt Benckiser LLC. Dr. Raymond W. Nims is employed by RMC Pharmaceutical Solutions, Inc. and received a fee from Reckitt Benckiser LLC for his role in authoring and editing the manuscript. Reckitt Benckiser LLC participated in the decision to publish.

Author details

M. Khalid Ijaz[1,2]*, Raymond W. Nims[3], Todd A. Cutts[4], Julie McKinney[1] and Charles P. Gerba[5]

1 Reckitt Benckiser, Montvale, NJ, USA

2 Medgar Evers College of the City University of New York (CUNY), Brooklyn, NY, USA

3 RMC Pharmaceutical Solutions, Inc., Longmont, CO, USA

4 Public Health Agency, Canada

5 University of Arizona, Tucson, AZ, USA

*Address all correspondence to: khalid.ijaz@rb.com

References

[1] World Health Organization. Prioritizing Diseases for Research and Development in Emergency Contexts. 2021. Available from: https://www.who.int/activities/prioritizing-diseases-for-research-and-development-in-emergency-contexts

[2] Nims RW, Zhou SS. Intra-family differences in efficacy of inactivation of small, non-enveloped viruses. Biologicals. 2016;**44**:456-462

[3] Zhou SS. Variability and relative order of susceptibility of non-enveloped viruses to chemical inactivation. In: Nims RW, Ijaz MK, editors. Disinfection of Viruses. London, UK: IntechOpen; 2021

[4] U.S. Environmental Protection Agency. Emerging Viral Pathogen Guidance for Antimicrobial Pesticides. 2021. Available from: https://www.epa.gov/pesticide-registration/emerging-viral-pathogen-guidance-antimicrobial-pesticides

[5] U.S. Environmental Protection Agency. Guidance to Registrants: Process for Making Claims against Emerging Viral Pathogens not on EPA-registered Disinfectant Labels. 2016. Available from: https://www.epa.gov/sites/default/files/2016-09/documents/emerging_viral_pathogen_program_guidance_final_8_19_16_001_0.pdf

[6] Spaulding EH. Chemical disinfection of medical and surgical materials. In: Block S, editor. Disinfection, Sterilization, and Preservation. 3rd ed. Philadelphia: Lea and Febiger; 1968

[7] Klein M, Deforest A. Principles of viral inactivation. In: Block SS, editor. Disinfection, Sterilization, and Preservation. 3rd ed. Philadelphia: Lea and Febiger; 1983. pp. 422-434

[8] Sattar SA. Hierarchy of susceptibility of viruses to environmental surface disinfectants: A predictor of activity against new and emerging viral pathogens. Journal of AOAC International. 2007;**90**(6):1655-1658

[9] Ijaz MK, Rubino JR. Should test methods for disinfectants use vertebrate virus dried on carriers to advance virucidal claims? Infection Control and Hospital Epidemiology. 2008;**29**(2): 192-194

[10] Ijaz MK, Sattar SA, Rubino JR, Nims RW, Gerba CP. Combating SARS-CoV-2: Leveraging microbicidal experiences with other emerging/re-emerging viruses. PeerJ. 2020;**8**:e9914. DOI: 10.7717/peerj.9914

[11] St. Georgiev V. Chapter 23: Defense against biological weapons (Biodefense). In: National Institute of Allergy and Infectious Diseases, NIH, Infectious Disease. Berlin: Springer; 2009. Available from: https://www.ncbi.nlm.nih.gov/pmc/articles/PMC7122899/pdf/978-1-60327-297-1_Chapter_23.pdf

[12] Chen Y, Liu Q, Guo D. Emerging coronaviruses: Genome structure, replication, and pathogenesis. Journal of Medical Virology. 2020;**92**:418-423

[13] Ang BSP, Lim TCC, Wang L. Nipah virus infection. Journal of Clinical Microbiology. 2018;**56**(6):e01875-e01817. DOI: 10.1128/JCM.01875-17

[14] Andersen KG, Rambaut A, Lipkin WI, Holmes EC, Garry RF. The proximal origin of SARS-CoV-2. Nature Medicine. 2020;**26**:450-455

[15] Ijaz MK, Nims RW, Zhou SS, Whitehead K, Srinivasan V, Kapes T, et al. Microbicidal actives with virucidal efficacy against SARS-CoV-2 and other beta- and alpha-coronaviruses and implications for future emerging coronaviruses and other enveloped

viruses. Scientific Reports. 2021;**11**:5626. DOI: 10.1038/s41598-021-84842-1

[16] Nims RW, Plavsic M. Physical inactivation of SARS-CoV-2 and other coronaviruses—A review. In: Nims RW, Ijaz MK, editors. Disinfection of Viruses. London, UK: IntechOpen; 2021

[17] Kindermann J, Karbiener M, Leydold SM, Knotzer S, Modrof J, Kreil TR. Virus disinfection for biotechnology applications: Different effectiveness on surface versus in suspension. Biologicals. 2020;**64**:1-9. DOI: 10.1016/j.biologicals.2020.02.002

[18] Mitchell SW, McCormick JB. Physicochemical inactivation of Lassa, Ebola, and Marburg viruses and effect on clinical laboratory analyses. Journal of Clinical Microbiology. 1984;**20**(3): 486-489

[19] Kochel TJ, Kocher GA, Ksiazek TG, Burans JP. Evaluation of TRIzol LS inactivation of viruses. ABSA International. 2017;**22**(2):52-55

[20] Lloyd G, Bowen ETW, Slade JHR. Physical and chemical methods of inactivating Lassa virus. The Lancet. 1982;**1**(8280):1046-1048

[21] Retterer C, Kenny T, Zamani R, Altamura LA, Kearney B, Jaissle J, et al. Strategies for validation of inactivation of viruses with Trizol LS® and formalin solutions. Applied Biosafety. 2020; **25**(2):74-82

[22] Al-Olayan EM, Mohamed AF, El-Khadraqy MF, Shebl RI, Yehia HM. An alternative inactivant for Rift Valley fever virus using cobra venom-derived L-amino oxidase, which is related to its immune potential. Brazilian Archives of Biology and Technology. 2016;**59**: e16160044. DOI: 10.1590/1678-4324-2016160044

[23] Kaschef AH. Inactivation of Rift Valley fever virus and related viral antigenicity and immunogenicity. Egyptian Journal of Medical Microbiology. 1996;**5**(3):459-464

[24] Hartman AL, Cole KS, Homer LC. Verification of inactivation methods for removal of biological materials from a biosafety level 3 select agent facility. Applied Biosafety. 2012;**17**(2):70-75

[25] United States Department of Agriculture. Foreign Animal Disease Preparedness & Response Plan. Henipavirus Standard Operating Procedures 1. Overview of Etiology and Ecology. 2013. Available from: https://www.aphis.usda.gov/animal_health/emergency_management/downloads/sop/sop_henipavirus_eande.pdf

[26] Gerlach M, Wolff S, Ludwig S, Schäfer W, Keiner B, Roth NJ, et al. Rapid SARS-CoV-2 inactivation by commonly available chemicals on inanimate surfaces. Journal of Hospital Infection. 2020;**106**:633-634

[27] Jahromi R, Mogharab V, Jahromi H, Avazpour A. Synergistic effects of anionic surfactants on coronavirus (SARS-CoV-2) virucidal efficiency of sanitizing fluids to fight COVID-19. Food and Chemical Toxicology. 2020; **145**:111702. DOI: 10.1016/j.fct.2020.111702

[28] Chin AWH, Chu JTS, Perera MRA, Hui KPY, Yen H-L, Chan MCW, et al. Stability of SARS-CoV-2 in different environmental conditions. The Lancet Microbe. 2020;**1**(1). DOI: 10.1016/S2666-5247(20)30003-3

[29] Xiling G, Yin C, Ling W, Xiaosong W, Jingjing F, Fang L, et al. In vitro inactivation of SARS-CoV-2 by commonly used disinfection products and methods. Scientific Reports. 2021; **11**:2418. DOI: 10.1038/s41598-021-82148-w

[30] Chan K-H, Sridhar S, Zhang RR, Chu H, Fung AY-F, Chan G, et al.

Factors affecting stability and infectivity of SARS-CoV-2. Journal of Hospital Infection. 2020;**106**:226-231

[31] Kratzel A, Todt D, V'kovski P, Steiner S, Gultom M, Thao TTN, et al. Inactivation of severe acute respiratory syndrome coronavirus 2 by WHO-recommended hand rub formulations and alcohols. Emerging Infectious Diseases. 2020;**26**(7). DOI: 10.3201/eid2607.200915

[32] Mantlo E, Rhodes T, Boutros J, Patterson-Fortin L, Evans A, Paessler S. In vitro efficacy of a copper iodine complex PPR disinfectant for SARS-CoV-2 inactivation. F1000Research. 2020;**9**:674. DOI: 10.12688/f1000research.24651.2

[33] Anderson DE, Sivalingam V, Kang AEZ, Ananthanarayanan A, Arumugam H, Jenkins TM, et al. Povidone-iodine demonstrates rapid in vitro virucidal activity against SARS-CoV-2, the virus causing COVID-19 disease. Infectious Diseases and Therapy. 2020;**9**:669-675

[34] Welch SR, Davies KA, Buczkowski H, Hettiarachchi N, Green N, Arnold U, et al. Analysis of inactivation of SARS-CoV-2 by specimen transport media, nucleic acid extraction reagents, detergents, and fixatives. Journal of Clinical Microbiology. 2020;**58**(11):e01713-e01720. DOI: 10.1128/JCM.01713-20

[35] Rabenau HF, Cinatl J, Morgenstern B, Bauer G, Preiser W, Doerr HW. Stability and inactivation of SARS coronavirus. Medical and Microbiological Immunology. 2005;**194**:1-6. DOI: 10.1007/s00430-004-0219-0

[36] Rabenau HF, Kampf G, Cinatl J, Doerr HW. Efficacy of various disinfectants against SARS coronavirus. Journal of Hospital Infection. 2005;**61**:107-111

[37] Kariwa H, Fujii N, Takashima I. Inactivation of SARS coronavirus by means of povidone-iodine, physical conditions and chemical reagents. Dermatology. 2006;**212**(Suppl. 1):119-123

[38] Hirose R, Bandou R, Ikegaya H, Watanabe N, Yoshida T, Daidoji T, et al. Disinfectant effectiveness against SARS-CoV-2 and influenza viruses present on human skin: Model based evaluation. Clinical Microbiology and Infection. 2021;**27**:1042.e1-1042.e4

[39] Leslie RA, Zhou SS, Macinga DR. Inactivation of SARS-CoV-2 by commercially available alcohol-based hand sanitizers. American Journal of Infection Control. 2021;**49**:401-402

[40] Siddharta A, Pfaender S, Vielle NJ, Dijkman R, Friesland M, Becker B, et al. Virucidal activity of World Health Organization-recommended formulations against enveloped viruses, including Zika, Ebola, and emerging coronaviruses. The Journal of Infectious Diseases. 2017;**215**:902-906

[41] Eggers M, Eickmann M, Zorn J. Rapid and effective virucidal activity of povidone-iodine products against Middle East respiratory syndrome coronavirus (MERS-CoV) and modified vaccinia Ankara (MVA). Infectious Disease and Therapy. 2015;**4**:491-501

[42] Patterson EI, Prince T, Anderson ER, Casas-Sanchez A, Smith SL, Cansado-Utrilla C, et al. Methods of inactivation of SARS-CoV-2 for downstream biological assays. Journal of Infectious Diseases. 2020;**222**:1462-1467

[43] Jureka AS, Silvas JA, Basler CE. Propagation, inactivation, and safety testing of SARS-CoV-2. Viruses. 2020;**12**(6):622. DOI: 10.3390/v120606222020

[44] Cook BWM, Cutts TA, Nikiforuk AM, Poliquin PG, Court DA, Srong JE, et al. Evaluating environmental persistence and disinfection of the Ebola

virus Makona variant. Viruses. 2015;**7**: 1975-1986

[45] Cook BWM, Cutts TA, Nikiforuk AM, Leung A, Kobasa D, Theriault SS. The disinfection characteristics of Ebola virus outbreak variants. Scientific Reports. 2016;**6**:38293. DOI: 10.1038/srep38293

[46] Smither SJ, Eastaugh L, Filone CM, Freeburger D, Herzog A, Lever MS, et al. Two-center evaluation of disinfectant efficacy against Ebola virus in clinical and laboratory matrices. Emerging Infectious Diseases. 2018; **24**(1):135-139

[47] Cutts TA, Robertson C, Theriault SS, Nims RW, Kasloff SB, Rubino JR, et al. Efficacy of microbicides for inactivation of Ebola-Makona virus on a non-porous surface: A targeted hygiene intervention for reducing virus spread. Scientific Reports. 2020;**10**:15247. DOI: 10.1038/s41598-020-71736-x

[48] Cutts TA, Kasloff SB, Krishnan J, Nims RW, Theriault SS, Rubino JR, et al. Comparison of the efficacy of disinfectant pre-impregnated wipes for decontaminating stainless steel carriers experimentally inoculated with Ebola virus and vesicular stomatitis virus. Frontiers in Public Health. 2021;**9**: 657443. DOI: 10.3389/pubh.2021.657443

[49] Smither S, Phelps A, Eastaugh L, Ngugi S, O'Brien L, Dutch A, et al. Effectiveness of four disinfectants against Ebola virus on different materials. Viruses. 2016;**8**:185. DOI: 10.3390/v8070185

[50] Cutts TA, Ijaz MK, Nims RW, Rubino JR, Theriault SS. Effectiveness of Dettol antiseptic liquid for inactivation of Ebola virus in suspension. Scientific Reports. 2019;**9**:6590. DOI: 10.1038/s41598-019-42386-5

[51] Eggers M, Eickmann M, Kowalski K, Zorn J, Reimer K. Povidone-iodine hand wash and hand rub products demonstrated excellent in vitro virucidal efficacy against Ebola virus and modified vaccinia virus Ankara, the new European test virus for enveloped viruses. BMC Infectious Diseases. 2015; **15**:375. DOI: 10.1186/s12879-015-1111-9

[52] Cutts TA, Nims RW, Theriault SS, Bruning E, Rubino JR, Ijaz MK. Hand hygiene: Virucidal efficacy of a liquid hand wash product against Ebola virus. Infection Prevention in Practice. 2021; **3**(1):100122. DOI: 10.1016/j.infpip.2021.100122

[53] Colavita F, Quartu S, Lalle E, Bordi L, Lapa D, Meschi S, et al. Evaluation of the inactivation effect of Triton X-100 on Ebola virus infectivity. Journal of Clinical Virology. 2017;**86**:27-30

[54] van Kampen JJA, Tintu A, Russcher H, Fraaij PLA, Reusken CBEM, Rijken M, et al. Ebola virus inactivation by detergents is annulled in serum. The Journal of Infectious Diseases. 2017;**216**: 859-866

[55] Wilde C, Chen Z, Kapes T, Chiosonne C, Lukula S, Suchmann D, et al. Inactivation and disinfection of Zika virus on a non-porous surface. Journal of Microbial and Biochemical Technology. 2016;**8**:5. DOI: 10.4172/1948-5948.1000319

[56] Müller JA, Harms M, Schubert A, Jansen S, Michel D, Mertens T, et al. Inactivation and environmental stability of Zika virus. Emerging Infectious Diseases. 2016;**22**(9):1685-1687

[57] Chida AS, Goldstein JM, Lee J, Tang X, Bedi K, Herzegh O, et al. Comparison of Zika virus inactivation methods for reagent production and disinfection methods. Journal of Virological Methods. 2021;**287**:114004

[58] Reynolds KA, Gerba CP, Pepper IL. Detection of infectious enteroviruses by integrated cell culture-PCR procedure.

Applied and Environmental Microbiology. 1996;**62**:1424-1427

[59] Killoran KE, Larson KL. Lassa Virus. Iowa State University; 2016. Available from: https://www.swinehealth.org/wp-content/uploads/2016/08/Lassa_Virus.pdf

[60] Spickler ER. Viral Hemorrhagic Fevers Caused by Arenaviruses. Iowa State University; 2010. Available from: http://www.cfsph.iastate.edu/DiseaseInfo/factsheets.php

[61] Spickler AR. Crimean-Congo Hemorrhagic Fever. Iowa State University Factsheet; 2019. Available from: https://www.cfsph.iastate.edu/Factsheets/pdfs/crimean_congo_hemorrhagic_fever.pdf

[62] Bartolini B, Gruber CEM, Koopmans M, Avšič T, Bino S, Christova I, et al. Laboratory management of Crimean-Congo haemorrhagic fever virus infections: Perspectives from two European networks. EuroSurveillance. 2019;**24**(5): 1800093. DOI: 10.2807/1560-7917.ES.2019.24.5.1800093

[63] Mukherjee S, Vincent CK, Jayasekera HW, Yekhe AS. Antiviral efficacy of personal care formulations against severe acute respiratory syndrome coronavirus 2. Infection, Disease & Health. 2021;**26**: 63-66

[64] Kumar M, Mazur S, Ork BL, Postnikova E, Hensley LE, Jahrling PB, et al. Inactivation and safety testing of Middle East respiratory syndrome coronavirus. Journal of Virological Methods. 2015;**223**:13-18. DOI: 10.1016/j.jviromet.2015.07.002

[65] Widera M, Westhaus S, Rabenau HF, Hoehl S, Bojkova D, Cinatl J Jr, et al. Evaluation of stability and inactivation methods of SARS-CoV-2 in context of laboratory settings. Medical Microbiology and Immunology. 2021; **210**:235-244

[66] Scheller C, Krebs F, Minkner R, Astner I, Gil-Moles M, Wätzig H. Physicochemical properties of SARS-CoV-2 for drug targeting, vaccine inactivation and attenuation, vaccine formulation and quality control. Electrophoresis. 2020;**41**(13-14): 1137-1151. DOI: 10.1002/elps.202000121

[67] Kampf G, Todt D, Pfaender S, Steinmann E. Persistence of coronaviruses on inanimate surfaces and their inactivation with biocidal agents. Journal of Hospital Infection. 2020;**104**: 246-251

[68] Mohan SV, Hemalatha M, Kopperi H, Ranjith I, Kumar AK. SARS-CoV-2 in environmental perspective: Occurrence, persistence, surveillance, inactivation, and challenges. Chemical Engineering Journal. 2021;**405**:126893. DOI: 10.1016/j.cej.2020.126893

[69] Quevedo-león R, Bastías-Montes JM, Espinoza-Tellez T, Ronceros B, Balic I, Muñoz O. Inactivation of coronaviruses in food industry: The use of inorganic and organic disinfectants, ozone, and UV radiation. Scientia Agropecuaria. 2020;**11**(2):257-266

[70] Weber DJ, Sickbert-Bennet EE, Kanamori H, Rutala WA. New and emerging infectious diseases (Ebola, Middle Eastern respiratory syndrome coronavirus, carbapenem-resistant Enterobacteriaceae, Candida auris): Focus on environmental survival and germicide susceptibility. American Journal of Infection Control. 2019;**47**: A29-A38

[71] Dev Kumar G, Mishra A, Dunn L, Townsend A, Oguadinma IC, Bright KR, et al. Biocides and novel antimicrobial agents for the mitigation of coronaviruses. Frontiers in Microbiology. 2020;**11**:1351. DOI: 0.3389/fmicb.2020.01351

[72] Schrank CL, Minbiole KPC, Wuest WM. Are quaternary ammonium compounds, the workhorse disinfectants, effective against severe acute respiratory syndrome coronavirus-2. ACS Infectious Diseases. 2020;**6**:1553-1557

[73] Sharafi SM, Ebrahimpour K, Nafez A. Environmental disinfection against COVID-19 in different areas of health care facilities: A review. Reviews in Environmental Health. 2021;**36**(2): 193-198

[74] Wolff MH, Sattar SA, Adegbunrin O, Tetro J. Environmental survival and microbicide inactivation of coronaviruses. In: Schmidt A, Wolff MH, Weber O, editors. Coronaviruses with Special Emphasis on First Insights Concerning SARS. Basel, Switzerland: Birkhäuser Verlag; 2005

[75] Kwok CS, Dashti M, Tafuro J, Nasiri M, Muntean E-A, Wong N, et al. Methods to disinfect and decontaminate SARS-CoV-2: A systematic review of in vitro studies. Therapeutic Advances in Infectious Disease. 2021;**8**:1-12. DOI: 10.1177/2049936121998548

[76] Ijaz MK, Nims RW, de Szalay S, Rubino JR. Soap, water, and severe acute respiratory syndrome coronavirus 2 (SARS-CoV-2): An ancient handwashing strategy for preventing dissemination of a novel virus. PeerJ. 2021;**9**:e12041. DOI: 10.7717/peerj.12041

[77] Iowa State University. Ebolavirus and Marburgvirus Infections. 2016. Available from: https://lib.dr.iastate.edu/cfsph_factsheets/50/

[78] World Health Organization. General Procedures for Inactivation of Potentially Infectious Samples with Ebola Virus and Other Highly Pathogenic Viral Agents. 2014. Available from: https://www.paho.org/hq/dmdocuments/2014/2014-cha-procedures-inactivation-ebola.pdf

[79] U.S. Department of Agriculture. Foreign Animal Disease Preparedness and Response Plan. Henipavirus Standard Operating Procedures: 1. Overview of Etiology and Ecology. 2013. Available from: https://www.aphis.usda.gov/animal_health/emergency_management/downloads/sop/sop_henipavirus_eande.pdf

[80] Verreault D, Moineau S, Duchaine C. Methods for sampling of airborne viruses. Microbiological and Molecular Biology Reviews. 2008;**72**(3):413-444

[81] Dancer SJ, Li Y, Hart A, Tang JW, Jones DL. What is the risk of acquiring SARS-CoV-2 from the use of public toilets? Science of the Total Environment. 2021;**792**:148341. DOI: 10.1016/j.scitotenv.2021.148341

[82] Ijaz MK, Zargar B, Wright KE, Rubino JR, Sattar SA. Generic aspects of the airborne spread of human pathogens indoors and emerging air decontamination technologies. American Journal of Infection Control. 2016;**44**:S109-S120

[83] Haines SR, Adams RI, Boor BE, Bruton TA, Downey J, Ferro AR, et al. Ten questions concerning the implications of carpet on indoor chemistry and microbiology. Building and Environment. 2020;**170**:106589. DOI: 10.1016/j.buildenv.2019.106589

[84] Stephens B, Azimi P, Thoemmes MS, Heidarinejad M, Allen JG, Gilbert JA. Microbial exchange via fomites and implications for human health. Current Pollution Reports. 2019;**5**:198-213

[85] National Institute of Allergy and Infectious Diseases (NIAID). Emerging Infectious Diseases/Pathogens Priority A List. 2018. Available from: https://www.niaid.nih.gov/research/emerging-infectious-diseases-pathogens

[86] National Institute of Allergy and Infectious Diseases (NIAID).

Coronaviruses. 2021. Available from: https://www.niaid.nih.gov/diseases-conditions/coronaviruses

[87] Morens DM, Fauci AS. Emerging pandemic diseases: How we got to COVID-19. Cell. 2020;**182**:1077-1092

[88] Schwartz DA. Prioritizing the continuing global challenges to emerging and reemerging viral infections. Frontiers in Virology. 2021;**1**: 701054. DOI: 10.3389/fviro.2021.701054

[89] World Health Organization. An R& D Blueprint for Action to Prevent Epidemics. 2017. Available from: h ttps://cdn.who.int/media/docs/default-source/blue-print/an-randd-blueprint-for-action-to-prevent-epidemics-update-2017.pdf?sfvrsn=4c31073a_1&d ownload=true

[90] Johns Hopkins University of Medicine. COVID-19 Data in Motion: Tuesday. 25 January 2022. Available from: https://coronavirus.jhu.edu/

[91] The World Health Organization (WHO). Classification of Omicron (B.1.1.529): SARS-CoV-2 Variant of Concern. Available from: https://www.who.int/news/item/26-11-2021-classification-of-omicron-(b.1.1.529)-sars-cov-2-variant-of-concern

[92] U.S. Centers for Disease Control and Prevention. SARS-CoV-2 Variant Classifications and Definitions. 2021. Available from: https://www.cdc.gov/coronavirus/2019-ncov/variants/variant-info.html

[93] Mandell RB, Flick R. Rift Valley fever virus: A real bioterror threat. Journal of Bioterrorism & Biodefense. 2011;**2**:2. DOI: 10.4172/2157-2526.1000108

[94] Blair PW, Kuhn JH, Pecor DB, Apanaskevich DA, Kortepeter MG, Cardile AP, et al. An emerging biothreat: Crimean-Congo hemorrhagic fever virus in Southern and Western Asia. American Journal of Tropical Medicine and Hygiene. 2019;**100**(1):16-23

[95] Sorvillo TE, Rodriguez SE, Hudson P, Carey M, Rodriguez LL, Spiropoulou CF, et al. Towards a sustainable One Health approach to Crimean-Congo haemorrhagic fever prevention: Focus areas and gaps in knowledge. Tropical Medicine and Infectious Disease. 2020; **5**:113. DOI: 10.3390/tropicalmed5030113

[96] Eggers M, Schwebke I, Suchomel M, Fotheringham V, Gebel J, Meyer B, et al. The European tiered approach for virucidal efficacy testing—Rationale for rapidly selecting disinfectants against emerging and re-emerging viral diseases. EuroSurveillance. 2021;**26**(3): 2000708. DOI: 10.2807/1560-7917.ES.2021.26.3.2000708

[97] Ijaz MK, Nims RW, McKinney J. SARS-CoV-2 mutational variants may represent a new challenge to society, but not to the virucidal armamentarium. Journal of Hospital Infection. 2021;**112**: 121-123

Chapter 6

Variability and Relative Order of Susceptibility of Non-Enveloped Viruses to Chemical Inactivation

Sifang Steve Zhou

Abstract

Viruses exhibit a marked variation in their susceptibilities to chemical and physical inactivation. Identifying a trend within these variations, if possible, could be valuable in the establishment of an effective and efficient infection control or risk mitigation strategy. It has been observed that non-enveloped viruses are generally less susceptible than enveloped viruses and that smaller sized viruses seem less susceptible than larger viruses. A theory of a "hierarchy" of pathogen susceptibility has been proposed and widely referenced. This concept provides a useful general guide for predicting the susceptibility of a newly emerged pathogen. It also serves as a theoretical basis for implementing a limited scale viral inactivation study that is to be extrapolated onto many other viruses. The hierarchy concept should be interpreted with caution since the actual viral inactivation efficacy may, in some cases, be different from the general prediction. The actual efficacy is dependent on the type of chemistry and application conditions. The order of susceptibility is not always fixed; and viruses within the same family or even the same genus may exhibit drastic differences. This chapter reviews viral inactivation data for several commonly used chemistries against non-enveloped viruses, highlighting the cases wherein the order of susceptibility varied or even flipped. Possible underlying mechanisms are also discussed.

Keywords: enveloped viruses, non-enveloped viruses, hierarchy of susceptibility, disinfection, viral inactivation, virucidal efficacy

1. Introduction

Bacteria, fungi (yeasts and molds), mycobacteria, prions, protozoa, and viruses are common pathogens infecting humans and animals. They typically exist within the host or in the environment. It has been observed that these microorganisms exhibit a notable difference in the natural survivability in the environment, as well as susceptibility to chemical and physical inactivation. For example, under ambient and dried conditions, human coronaviruses seem to lose their infectivity in a matter of several hours to several days [1], whereas endospores and prions may remain infectious for years to decades or even indefinitely [2, 3].

As more and more data have become available regarding the survivability and susceptibility of pathogens to microbicides, it has been observed that the pathogens seem to demonstrate an order of susceptibility to chemical and physical inactivation. E. H. Spaulding first proposed a classification system for the sterilization and disinfection of medical instruments based on the infection risk in 1939 [4]. On the basis of this classification, the concept of a hierarchy of pathogen susceptibility was proposed, in which microorganisms are placed into several groups and ranked from least susceptible to most susceptible. In this hierarchy concept, bacterial spores were ranked the least susceptible, followed by mycobacteria, non-enveloped viruses, fungi, vegetative bacteria, and enveloped viruses. The susceptibility hierarchy was also believed to be related to the biochemical and biophysical characteristics of a pathogen [5, 6].

This hierarchy concept has been slightly modified and expanded over the years. For example, prions were added and considered less susceptible to inactivation by microbicides than bacterial spores; small non-enveloped viruses were considered less susceptible than large non-enveloped viruses; and the order between mycobacteria and small non-enveloped viruses was sometimes reversed (**Figure 1**) [7–10]. Additionally, it has been suggested that the hierarchy concept may be applied either "vertically" (i.e., ranking of susceptibility *between* classes of pathogens) and/or "horizontally" (i.e., ranking of susceptibility *within* a class of pathogens) [11].

The hierarchy concept has been quite useful for enabling scientists to better understand the innate difference among various types of pathogens. In the case of newly emerged pathogens, especially, the hierarchy concept has helped stakeholders design and implement a disinfection strategy swiftly with a reasonable level of confidence. The concept also helps the contaminant control for food, pharmaceutical, and biopharmaceutical products, as it is impractical to test every possible contaminating pathogen, and a robust infectivity assay system may be lacking for certain pathogens (e.g., hepatitis E virus).

Despite its usefulness, the hierarchy concept should be interpreted with caution, as it may oversimply the differences and trending of pathogen susceptibilities. Further examination and refinement of the concept may be necessary; and several important questions should be answered. For example, how often do exceptions to the hierarchy occur and what are the underlying reasons? Could a trending be specific to a given type of chemistry? Is the hierarchy the same between susceptibility to both chemical and physical inactivation? Why do pathogens in the same

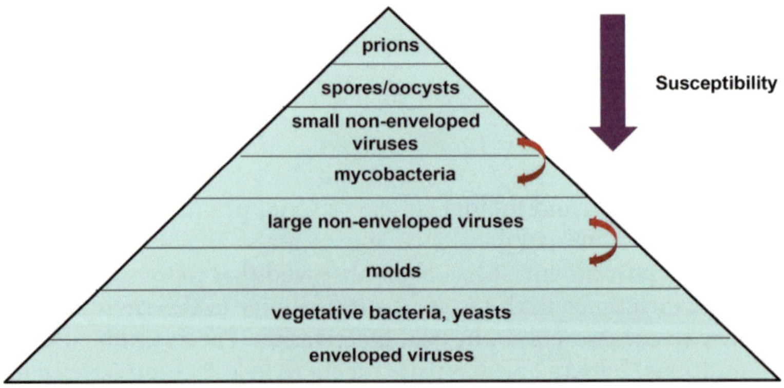

Figure 1.
Proposed hierarchy of susceptibility of pathogens to microbicides. Note: slightly different versions of the hierarchy concept have been proposed in the literature. Mycobacteria have been placed above small non-enveloped viruses, and molds have been placed above large non-enveloped viruses in certain versions. In some versions, the small and large non-enveloped viruses are combined; and yeasts and molds may be combined.

group, or even the same family or genus, sometimes exhibit striking differences in susceptibility? Is there a way to identify and separate reliable/consistent trending versus blurred/variable trending? A deeper look at the efficacy data for various types of microbicidal actives, especially for non-enveloped viruses, may help stakeholders understand the scope, reliability, and limitation of the hierarchy concept so that it can be best utilized.

This chapter reviews the inactivation efficacy data from the literature against non-enveloped viruses for several commonly used types of chemistries, either in formulated or unformulated form, in an effort to generate a separate relative order of susceptibility among these non-enveloped viruses for each type of chemistry and to differentiate consistent versus variable trending. Physical inactivation approaches are not covered in this chapter, although a significant degree of variation also exists for physical treatments. It is not clear that the physical inactivation approaches, in general, are governed by the same hierarchy to susceptibility as is observed for chemical inactivation approaches [12].

2. Common families of mammalian non-enveloped viruses

Currently, there are a total of 21 families of viruses (including enveloped and non-enveloped) identified for humans [13], which represent only a small part of the entire paradigm of viruses in nature, whose host ranges extend from vertebrates to plants to bacteria. The most common families of non-enveloped viruses for humans and animals include *Adenoviridae, Astroviridae, Caliciviridae, Circoviridae, Hepeviridae, Papillomaviridae, Parvoviridae, Picornaviridae, Polyomaviridae,* and *Reoviridae.* The genome structure, size of viral particle, and some representative viruses for each viral family are presented in **Table 1**.

Among these, the *Adenoviridae and Reoviridae* families of viruses are generally considered large, non-enveloped viruses. Other non-enveloped viruses are generally considered small, non-enveloped viruses, although it should be noted that the particle sizes of *Papillomaviruses* and *Polyomaviruses* are notably larger than those for the rest of the small non-enveloped virus group (**Table 1**).

It is worth noting that viruses are typically classified taxonomically on the basis of virion properties (size, shape, envelope, physical, and chemical properties, etc.), genome organization, replication mechanism, antigenic properties, and biological properties [13–15]. The final classification is a combined consideration of these properties. However, the stability and susceptibility to inactivation of a virus may not relate to all of these properties and, as such, may not always align with the taxonomic classification system. For example, the susceptibility of a virus to surfactants may primarily be related to the envelope of the virion and not related to the genome structure or mode of replication.

The susceptibilities of non-enveloped viruses to chemicals have been found to be highly variable and somewhat hard to predict, since they do not always agree with the hierarchy concept. For example, according to the hierarchy concept as modified by Sattar [8], small non-enveloped viruses should be less susceptible than large non-enveloped viruses. Additionally, if there is a fixed hierarchy, all small non-enveloped viruses should either display similar levels of susceptibility or should demonstrate a definitive trend of relative susceptibility, regardless of the type of microbicide. Based on the literature, neither of these predictions appear to hold in every case. The relative order of susceptibility seems chemistry-dependent; and sometimes viruses within the same family or even genus have been found to exhibit unequivocal differences in their susceptibilities (reviewed in [16]). Any trending or

Family	Example virus	Abbreviation	Genus	Genome	Size (nm)
Adenoviridae	Adenovirus type 2	AdV-2	*Mastadenovirus*	ds DNA	70–90
	Adenovirus type 5	AdV-5	*Mastadenovirus*	ds DNA	70–90
	Adenovirus type 8	AdV-8	*Mastadenovirus*	ds DNA	70–90
Astroviridae	Human astrovirus	HAstV	*Mamastrovirus*	ss RNA	28–35
Caliciviridae	Feline calicivirus	FCV	*Vesivirus*	ss RNA	28–40
	Human norovirus	HuNoV	*Norovirus*	ss RNA	28–40
	Murine norovirus	MNV	*Norovirus*	ss RNA	28–40
	Tulane virus	TuV	*Recovirus*	ss RNA	28–40
Circoviridae	Porcine circovirus	PCV	*Circovirus*	ss DNA	~17
Hepeviridae	Hepatitis E virus	HEV	*Orthohepevirus*	ss DNA	32–34
Papillomaviridae	Human papillomavirus	HPV	*Papillomavirus*	ds DNA	50–60
Parvoviridae	Bovine parvovirus	BPV	*Bocaparvovirus*	ss DNA	20–28
	Canine parvovirus	CPV	*Protoparvovirus*	ss DNA	20–25
	Human parvovirus B19	B19V	*Erythroparvovirus*	ss DNA	23–26
	Minute virus of mice	MVM (MMV)	*Protoparvovirus*	ss DNA	20–25
	Porcine parvovirus	PPV	*Protoparvovirus*	ss DNA	20–25
Picornaviridae	Bovine enterovirus	BEV	*Enterovirus*	ss RNA	30–32
	Coxsackievirus	Cox	*Enterovirus*	ss RNA	30–32
	Echovirus 11	Echo11	*Enterovirus*	ss RNA	30–32
	Encephalomyocarditis virus	EMCV	*Cardiovirus*	ss RNA	30–32
	Enterovirus 71	EV-71	*Enterovirus*	ss RNA	30–32
	Enterovirus D68	EV-D68	*Enterovirus*	ss RNA	30–32
	Foot and mouth disease virus	FMDV	*Aphthovirus*	ss RNA	30–32
	Hepatitis A virus	HAV	*Hepatovirus*	ss RNA	30–32
	Poliovirus type 1	PV1	*Enterovirus*	ss RNA	30–32
	Rhinovirus	RV	*Enterovirus*	ss RNA	30–32
	Seneca Valley virus	SVV	*Senecavirus*	ss RNA	30–32
Polyomaviridae	Bovine polyomavirus	BPyV	*Polyomavirus*	ds DNA	40–50
	Simian virus 40	SV40	*Betapolyomavirus*	ds DNA	40–50
Reoviridae	Bluetongue virus	BTV	*Orbivirus*	ds RNA	60–80
	Reovirus type 3	REO-3	*Orthoreovirus*	ds RNA	60–80
	Rotavirus	Rota	*Rotavirus*	ds RNA	60–80

ss *single-stranded;* ds *double-stranded.*

Table 1.
Common families of human and animal non-enveloped viruses.

hierarchy, therefore, must be reviewed in the context of the type of chemistry, and it should not be assumed that non-enveloped viruses within the same family or genus will always display similar susceptibilities to a given microbicide.

3. Overview of chemical viral inactivation approaches

Viral inactivation may be achieved by chemical and/or physical methods. The subset of chemicals commonly used for inactivation of non-enveloped viruses includes alcohols, oxidizers, halogen compounds, quaternary ammonium compounds, phenolics, aldehydes, acids, and alkalines [17–19]. These differ with respect to efficacy, stability, toxicity, material or surface compatibility, cost, and sensitivity to organic soil load. Soil load is a term used to signify an organic matrix used to challenge the inactivating efficacy of a microbicide. It is intended to mimic secretions or excretions in which the virus would be released from an infected person or animal. Some chemistries (e.g., sodium hypochlorite, phenolics, and aldehydes) are mostly used for environmental or medical device disinfection. Other chemistries (e.g., ethanol) are more commonly used for hand hygiene, while some others (e.g., quaternary ammonium compounds) may be used for both environmental disinfection and skin antisepsis (**Table 2**).

The virucidal efficacy of a product is not only determined by the type and concentration of the chemical, but is also heavily influenced by the formulation, pH, exposure (contact or dwell) time, organic soil load, temperature, and surface characteristics (as applicable), etc. [10, 20–22]. Given the differences between various testing methods, as well as the intrinsic variability of viral infectivity (titration) assays, a general conclusion on the efficacy of a particular type of active ingredient will be enhanced if the efficacy is derived from multiple sets of data and under various application conditions (such as the concentration of the microbicidal active(s), contact time, formulation matrix (as applicable), and organic soil load, etc.) Additionally, in order best to explore the relative ranking of susceptibility between viruses, or the lack thereof, efficacy data from side-by-side studies wherein the same test methodologies and conditions were used would be preferable. Care should be taken when comparing data from different studies, especially if the formulations, test methods, and test conditions were different.

4. Inactivation of non-enveloped viruses by alcohols

Alcohols, primarily ethanol and isopropanol, are widely used for hand hygiene and environmental disinfection, and their efficacies against bacteria and viruses have been extensively studied [23–25]. Ethanol at a concentration of 70–90% and isopropanol at 70% have been broadly shown to be effective against enveloped viruses; however, their efficacies against non-enveloped viruses are much more variable.

The trending of the degree of susceptibility of non-enveloped viruses to ethanol and isopropanol is generally clearer and more consistent than it is for many other types of chemistries, thanks to the large amount of data in the literature. The relative ranking of susceptibility of non-enveloped viruses seems to differ between ethanol and isopropanol; and the ranking does not appear to align well with the classical virological taxonomy.

For ethanol, parvoviruses and the polyomavirus simian virus 40 have low susceptibility, while rotavirus (a reovirus) is susceptible (**Table 3**). Viruses in the *Picornaviridae* family display clear differences in their susceptibilities to ethanol; and even viruses within the same genus display marked differences. For example, hepatitis A virus and human enterovirus 71 are much less susceptible than rhinovirus; and poliovirus, foot-and-mouth disease virus, and coxsackie virus seem to exhibit intermediate levels of susceptibility compared with the aforementioned viruses. The viral family *Caliciviridae* also has shown drastic differences among family members in the susceptibility to ethanol. Murine norovirus is quite susceptible to ethanol, whereas

Class	Chemical	Typical conc.	Usage	Mechanism of viral inactivation	Sensitivity to soil load
Alcohols	Ethanol	50–95%	Disinfection; Antisepsis	Protein denaturation	+
	Isopropanol	70–90%	Disinfection	Protein denaturation	+
Oxidizers	Sodium hypochlorite	0.01–0.5%	Disinfection	Protein/genome damage	++
	Chlorine dioxide	0.1–1 mg/L	Disinfection; Water treatment	Protein/genome damage	—
	Hydrogen peroxide	0.1–10%	Disinfection; Antisepsis	Lipid/protein/genome damage	+
	Hypochlorous acid	0.002–0.1%	Disinfection; Water treatment	Protein/genome damage	++
	Peracetic acid	0.01–1%	Disinfection; Sterilization	Protein denaturation	—
	Povidone-iodine	0.02–8%	Disinfection; Antisepsis	Protein/genome damage	++
	Chlorohexidine	0.02–0.2%	Antisepsis	Protein denaturation	+
QAC	BKC, DDAC, etc.	0.01–0.2%	Disinfection	Lipid/protein damage	+
Low pH	Acids	≤ pH 4	Sanitization; Biomanufacturing	Capsid/protein damage	—
High pH	NaOH, etc.	≥ pH 10	Disinfection; Tissue processing	Capsid/genome damage	—
Aldehydes	Glutaraldehyde	0.02–2%	HLD; Sterilization	Crosslinking/protein & genome damage	—
	Formaldehyde	0.1–5%	Disinfection/ Preservation	Alkylating/protein & genome damage	—
	OPA	0.02–2%	HLD; Sterilization	Crosslinking/protein damage	—
Phenolics	Phenylphenol, etc.	0.05–5%	Disinfection	Protein damage	—

Abbreviations used: BKC, benzalkonium chloride; Conc, concentration; DDAC, didecyldimethylammonium chloride; HLD, high-level disinfection; NaOH, sodium hydroxide; OPA, ortho-phthaldehyde; QAC, quaternary ammonium compounds.

Table 2.
Common types of chemistries used for non-enveloped viral inactivation.

feline calicivirus, human norovirus, and Tulane virus are significantly more difficult to inactivate with ethanol. The *Adenoviridae* is another non-enveloped virus family that has shown intrafamily differences, wherein adenovirus 5 is rather susceptible but adenovirus 2 and adenovirus 8 are much less susceptible. The relative order of susceptibility between murine norovirus (a small, non-enveloped virus) and adenovirus types 2 and 8 (two large, non-enveloped viruses) clearly conflicts with the simplified hierarchy concept (**Figure 1**).

Interestingly, the above order of susceptibility does not appear to hold the same for isopropanol (**Table 3**). For example, the polyomavirus simian virus 40 is much more susceptible to isopropanol than many other non-enveloped viruses; and poliovirus appears to display a lower susceptibility, similar to that of hepatitis A virus and human enterovirus 71. Murine norovirus is still more susceptible than

Virus[a]	Method	Soil/Matrix[b]	Log$_{10}$ Reduction after				References
			30 s	1 min	5 min	10 min	
70% Ethanol							
PPV	Stainless steel	Erythrocytes + BSA		0.3		0.6	[26]
MVM	Stainless steel	Erythrocytes + BSA		0.3		0.7	[26]
HEV71	Suspension test	Medium				< 1	[27]
HAV	Suspension test	Medium			0.4		[28]
HAV	Suspension test	20% fecal			0.4		[28]
HuNoV	Suspension test	20% stool		<0.5			[29]
TuV	Suspension test	Medium				<0.5	[30]
PV1	Suspension test	20% fecal			0.3		[28]
PV1	Suspension test	Medium			0.4		[31]
PV1	Glass	Medium		2.3	1.0	5.0	[31]
PV1	Stainless steel	Erythrocytes + BSA		2.1		1.8	[26]
PV1	Suspension test	Medium			4		[28]
FCV	Suspension test	Medium			0.5	2.6	[32]
FCV	Suspension test	Medium			1.7	2.2	[30]
AdV-8	Suspension test	Medium			1.9		[33]
AdV-5	Stainless steel	Erythrocytes + BSA		2.4		>4.1	[26]
AdV-5	Stainless steel	Medium			~5		[34]
MNV	Suspension test	Medium			> 3.6		[32]
MNV	Suspension test	Medium			5		[30]
Rotavirus	Suspension test	Medium			> 3.1		[28]
75% Ethanol							
RV86	Filter	Medium			>5		[35]
80% Ethanol							
CPV	Stainless steel	Medium			0.1		[36]
SV40	Suspension test	Medium				<1	[37]
FCV	Suspension test	Medium		1.3			[38]
FMDV	Suspension test	Medium			2.3		[39]
PV1	Glass	Medium		2.9	2.9	5.4	[31]
PV1	Suspension test	Medium		4.2			[40]
PV1	Suspension test	Medium		4.2			[41]
70% Isopropanol							
TuV	Suspension test	Medium				<0.5	[30]
FCV	Suspension test	Medium				<0.5	[30]
FCV	Suspension test	Medium		0.1	0.2		[32]
HEV71	Suspension test	Medium				<1	[27]
PV1	Suspension test	medium				<1	[37]
PV1	Glass	Medium		1.2	1.3	1.0	[31]
AdV-5	Stainless steel	Medium			~1		[34]

Virus[a]	Method	Soil/Matrix[b]	Log$_{10}$ Reduction after				References
			30 s	1 min	5 min	10 min	
AdV-8	Suspension test	Medium		2.0			[33]
MNV	Suspension test	Medium		2.6	>2.6		[32]
MNV	Suspension test	Medium		1.8	3.1		[30]
SV40	Suspension test	Medium				>4	[37]
Rotavirus	Suspension test	Medium		> 4			[42]

*[a]See **Table 1** for abbreviations used for viruses.*
[b]BSA, bovine serum albumin; medium, culture medium; RT, room temperature.
Entries in purple font indicate results from undiluted or diluted formulations with the indicated microbicidal active ingredients.

Table 3.
Efficacy of alcohols against non-enveloped viruses.

feline calicivirus to isopropanol, but not as susceptible as simian virus 40 or rotavirus. The apparent difference between adenovirus 5 and adenovirus 8 that has been observed for ethanol has not been observed for isopropanol.

5. Inactivation of non-enveloped viruses by oxidizers

An oxidizer or oxidizing agent is a chemical that has the ability to oxidize other molecules, i.e., to accept their electrons. Common oxidizing agents used for disinfection, sterilization, or antisepsis include hydrogen peroxide, peracetic acid, ozone, and halogen-containing compounds such as sodium hypochlorite (bleach), hypochlorous acid, povidone-iodine, chlorohexidine, and chlorine dioxide, etc. These compounds can react with and alter the proteins and nucleic acids of non-enveloped viruses and render them noninfectious. Oxidizers comprise a large group of chemicals, and the relative order of susceptibility of non-enveloped viruses to oxidizers seems to vary by specific type of active ingredient (**Table 4**).

Parvoviruses are generally among the least susceptible viruses to various types of oxidizers, including sodium hypochlorite, hydrogen peroxide, and peracetic acid. However, for sodium hypochlorite, minute virus of mice appears to be more susceptible than porcine parvovirus and canine parvovirus. All picornaviruses appear to exhibit a similar degree of susceptibility to sodium hypochlorite; but within the family of *Caliciviridae*, feline calicivirus appears to be more susceptible than murine norovirus. Both adenovirus and rotavirus are susceptible to sodium hypochlorite.

The trending for hydrogen peroxide seems more complex than that for sodium hypochlorite. For example, there seems a higher level of variability within the *Picornaviridae* family. Rhinovirus is quite susceptible to hydrogen peroxide, whereas hepatitis A virus is much less susceptible. Poliovirus seems to be more susceptible than hepatitis A virus but less susceptible than rhinovirus. Similar to the case for sodium hypochlorite, feline calicivirus seems more susceptible than murine norovirus to hydrogen peroxide. Interestingly, adenovirus and rotavirus, two larger non-enveloped viruses, seem to be less susceptible than rhinovirus, a smaller virus, to inactivation by hydrogen peroxide. This is another case where the size of viral particle alone does not appear to dictate the level of susceptibility to a microbicide.

For peracetic acid, hepatitis A virus also seems less susceptible than poliovirus. Both feline calicivirus and murine norovirus are susceptible to peracetic acid and so is adenovirus.

Virus[a]	Method	Soil/Matrix[b]	Log$_{10}$ Reduction after				References
			≤ 1 min	2 min	5 min	10 min	
Sodium hypochlorite, 0.05%							
FCV	Suspension test	Medium	3				[29]
FCV	Suspension test	20% stool	0.5				[29]
MNV	Suspension test	Medium	3				[29]
MNV	Suspension test	20% stool	0.0				[29]
Sodium hypochlorite, 0.1%							
CPV	Stainless steel	90% plasma				< 1	[43]
MNV	Stainless steel	10% stool				< 1	[44]
MNV	Stainless steel	medium			1.4		[30]
TuV	Stainless steel	medium			1.2		[30]
CPV	Stainless steel	5% serum				5	[43]
FCV	Stainless steel	medium			5.3		[30]
FCV	Stainless steel	10% stool				~2	[44]
HAV	Stainless steel	5% serum	5				[43]
HAV	Stainless steel	90% plasma	<1			5	[43]
HAV	Suspension test	PBS/20% fecal				4	[28]
PV1	Suspension test	PBS/20% fecal				4	[28]
PV1	Glass	Medium	0.9			2.2	[31]
RV14	Stainless steel	Mucin				2.5	[45]
Sodium hypochlorite, 0.25%							
PPV	Stainless steel	Erythrocytes + BSA	0.6			1.0	[26]
MVM	Stainless steel	Erythrocytes + BSA	3.0			4.4	[26]
PV1	Stainless steel	Erythrocytes + BSA	2.8			4.5	[26]
PV1	Glass	Medium	3.1		>4	5.3	[31]
AdV-5	Stainless steel	Erythrocytes + BSA	4				[26]
Sodium hypochlorite, ~0.3%							
Cox A16	Glass	Medium			> 3		[46]
EV71	Glass	Medium			> 3		[46]
Sodium hypochlorite, 0.5%							
MNV	Stainless steel	10% stool		< 1		~3.2	[44]
MVM	Stainless steel	Medium	1.2		2.2		[47]
MVM	Suspension test	Medium	2.5		> 4		[47]
FCV	Stainless steel	10% stool		3.2		> 5	[44]
Hydrogen peroxide, ~0.05%							
HAV	Stainless steel	Medium				~3.8	[47]
MVM	Stainless steel	Medium				>4.6	[47]
Hydrogen peroxide, ~0.1%							
PV1	Glass	Medium		0.4		0.9	[16]
RV14	Glass	Medium		>4.9			[16]

Virus[a]	Method	Soil/Matrix[b]	Log$_{10}$ Reduction after				References
			≤1 min	2 min	5 min	10 min	
FCV	Suspension test	Medium				>3	[48]
Hydrogen peroxide, 1%							
Rotavirus	Stainless steel	Non-purified virus			1		[49]
Rotavirus	Stainless steel	Purified virus			>3		[49]
MNV	Stainless steel	Medium		1.1	2.0		[50]
Hydrogen peroxide, 3%							
PV1	Suspension test	Medium		<0.5	<0.5		[31]
PV1	Glass	Medium		2.1	2.4	3.5	[31]
Hydrogen peroxide, 7.5%							
PPV	Stainless steel	Erythrocytes + BSA				0.5	[26]
MVM	Stainless steel	Erythrocytes + BSA				1.5	[26]
PV1	Stainless steel	Erythrocytes + BSA				3.9	[26]
AdV-5	Stainless steel	Erythrocytes + BSA				2.3	[26]
Peracetic acid, 100 ppm							
HAV	Washing[c]	Medium		<1			[51]
FCV	Washing[c]	Medium		3.2			[51]
MNV	Washing[c]	Medium		2.3			[51]
Peracetic acid, 500 ppm							
MNV	Suspension test	Medium	~3				[52]
Peracetic acid, 640 ppm							
HAV	Suspension test	Medium				~3	[53]
PV	Suspension test	Medium				>3	[53]
Peracetic acid, 1000 ppm							
CPV	Stainless steel	BSA			1.6		[34]
MVM	Stainless steel	BSA			2.3-2.9		[34]
PPV	Stainless steel	BSA			3.8-5.5		[34]
AdV-5	Stainless steel	BSA			4.9-5.8		[34]

*[a]See **Table 1** for abbreviations used for viruses.*
bBSA, bovine serum albumin; PBS, phosphate buffered saline; medium, culture medium; RT, room temperature.
[c]Viral-inoculated lettuce was washed with PAA solution for a defined period of time.
Entries in purple font indicate results from undiluted original or diluted formulations with microbicidal active ingredients.

Table 4.
Efficacy of oxidizers against non-enveloped viruses.

6. Inactivation of non-enveloped viruses by quaternary ammonium compounds

Quaternary ammonium compounds (QAC) are widely used as active ingredients for disinfectants. Among the advantages of QAC are good stability, dual function of disinfection and cleaning, surface activity, low toxicity, and lack of odor, etc. The potential limitation in the microbicidal efficacy and possible effect in promoting antimicrobial resistance of QAC have also been discussed in the literature [54, 55].

Virus[a]	Method	Soil/matrix[b]	Log_{10} reduction after				References
			30 s	1 min	10 min	60 min	
QAC 0.05%							
PPV	Stainless steel	Erythrocytes + BSA			0.4		[26]
MVM	Stainless steel	Erythrocytes + BSA			0.5		[26]
PV1	Stainless steel	Erythrocytes + BSA			0.5		[26]
AdV-5	Stainless steel	Erythrocytes + BSA			1.8		[26]
Rotavirus	Suspension	Medium			>5		[56]
QAC 0.1%							
AdV-8	Suspension test	Medium				1.0-1.8	[57]
AdV-5	Suspension test	Medium				3.7-5.3	[57]
TuV	Suspension test	Medium		<0.5			[30]
QAC 0.2%							
PV1	Suspension test	BSA/yeast extract		0.0			[58]
AdV-25	Suspension test	BSA/yeast extract		0.3			[58]
Cox A11	Suspension test	BSA/yeast extract		>5.1			[58]
QAC 0.9%							
FCV	Suspension test	Medium	<0.5				[29]
MNV	Suspension test	Medium	<0.5				[29]
Mixed QACs							
FCV	Suspension test	Medium		0.5	2.6		[44]
Rhinovirus	Glass	Medium	>3.0		>3.3		[16]

*[a]See **Table 1** for abbreviations used for viruses.*
[b]BSA, bovine serum albumin; medium, culture medium; QAC, quaternary ammonium compound.
Entries in purple font indicate results from original or diluted formulations with microbicidal active ingredients.

Table 5.
Efficacy of QAC against non-enveloped viruses.

Quaternary ammonium compounds are generally efficacious on most vegetative bacteria and enveloped viruses. Their efficacies against non-enveloped viruses, however, are generally much weaker. Nevertheless, several non-enveloped viruses, such as rotavirus, rhinovirus, and coxsackievirus A11, have been shown to be susceptible to QAC. The susceptibility levels among the *Adenoviridae* family of viruses seem to vary, with adenovirus 8 displaying less susceptibility than adenovirus 5. Both feline calicivirus and murine norovirus display low susceptibility to QAC (**Table 5**). The relative order of susceptibility of non-enveloped viruses to QAC does not seem to align well with the relative size of the virions; and the efficacy of QAC is often dependent on the product formulation.

7. Inactivation of non-enveloped viruses by low pH and high pH

Acids and alkalines, either used alone or in combination with other active ingredients in formulated products, can be an effective means for viral inactivation. Acids may be used for disinfection, sanitization, textile or face mask pretreatment, or viral clearance during biopharmaceutical manufacturing. Alkalines may also be used for disinfection, sanitization, and viral clearance during biopharmaceutical manufacturing and can be effective against even the least susceptible of pathogens, the prions [58].

It has been widely reported that a low-pH treatment (typically at pH 4 and below) can effectively inactivate most enveloped viruses, although some enveloped viruses, such as bovine viral diarrhea virus, still exhibit a relatively low susceptibility to this treatment pH [22]. The range of susceptibilities of non-enveloped viruses to low pH seems quite scattered and often goes against the "conventional wisdom" that non-enveloped viruses are not susceptible to acidic pH (**Table 6**). For instance, in the

Virus[a]	Method	Soil/Matrix[b]	Log_{10} Reduction after				References
			20 min	30 min	45 min	1–2 hr	
pH < 2							
REO-3	Suspension test	Medium				1–3	[59]
PCV	Suspension test	Medium				>3	[60]
pH 2.0							
MVM	Suspension test	Medium				<1	[61]
MNV	Suspension test	Medium		<0.5			[30]
TuV	Suspension test	Medium		<0.5			[30]
PARV4	Suspension test	Medium				2–3	[61]
B19V	Suspension test	Medium				> 4	[61]
FCV	Suspension test	Medium		6.3			[30]
FCV	Suspension test	Medium		>5			[62]
pH ~ 2.6							
PV	Suspension test	Medium		<1			[63]
PV	Suspension test	Medium				<1	[64]
HAV	Suspension test	Medium				<1	[64]
pH 3.0							
MNV	Suspension test	Medium		<0.5			[30]
TuV	Suspension test	Medium		<0.5			[30]
Cox A9	Suspension test	Medium	<1				[65]
FCV	Suspension test	Medium		~3			[30]
FCV	Suspension test	Medium		~4.7			[62]
RV	Suspension test	Medium	>3				[65]
FMDV	Suspension test	Medium	>3				[65]
pH 4.0							
MVM	Suspension test	Medium				<1	[66]
EV71	Suspension test	Medium			<1		[67]
EV-D68	Suspension test	Medium			~4–5	<5	[67]
B19V	Suspension test	Medium					[66]

[a]*See **Table 1** for abbreviations used for viruses.*
[b]*Medium, culture medium.*

Table 6.
Efficacy of low pH against non-enveloped viruses.

family of *Parvoviridae*, human parvovirus B19 has been found to be markedly susceptible to low pH (completely inactivated after 1–2 h treatment at pH 4), whereas animal parvoviruses, such as minute virus of mice, are not inactivated at all under the same conditions. Interestingly, another human parvovirus (type 4) appears to be less susceptible than B19, but more susceptible than minute virus of mice.

The *Picornaviridae* family also exhibits disparity with respect to susceptibility to low pH. For instance, hepatitis A virus, poliovirus, human enterovirus 71, and coxsackievirus A9 display low susceptibility (less than 1-$\log_{10}$ reduction at pH 3–4 for 1–2 h), whereas rhinovirus, foot-and-mouth disease virus, and enterovirus EV-D68 are highly susceptible (more than 4-$\log_{10}$ reduction or complete inactivation at pH 3–4 after 20–45 min). Note that human enterovirus 71, coxsackievirus A9, rhinovirus, and enterovirus EV-D68 are all members of the same genus (*Enterovirus*).

Feline calicivirus and murine norovirus in the family *Caliciviridae* represent another interesting and convincing example that not all viruses within the same family exhibit the same degree of susceptibility. As an example, feline calicivirus is susceptible to low pH, whereas murine norovirus is much less susceptible. Rotavirus and reovirus (family *Reoviridae*) also display low susceptibility to low pH. The low susceptibility of murine norovirus and rotavirus to low pH may not be a surprise, since these viruses naturally exist in the digestive track, which has an acidic environment. Feline calicivirus, on the other hand, acts more like a respiratory virus.

Viruses, both enveloped and non-enveloped, are generally susceptible to high pH. At an environment of pH 12 or above, most if not all non-enveloped viruses would be inactivated, with extent depending both on temperature and contact time. Reovirus, simian virus 40, hepatitis A virus, canine parvovirus, poliovirus, murine norovirus, and Tulane virus seem to be less susceptible than minute virus of mice, feline calicivirus, adenovirus, rotavirus, and foot-and-mouth disease virus. It may be worth noting that the order of susceptibility to high pH seems to be in discord with the hierarchy concept by the greatest degree: in this case, an enveloped virus, bovine viral diarrhea virus, seems to be less susceptible than most, if not all, non-enveloped viruses [22]; parvoviruses are not necessarily less susceptible than many other non-enveloped viruses; and the size of the viral particle does not seem to matter much with regard to the degree of susceptibility (**Table 7**).

Virus[a]	**Method**	**Soil/Matrix**[b]	**$\log_{10}$ Reduction after**				**References**
			≤1 min	**10 min**	**30 min**	**1 hr**	
pH 10							
MNV	Suspension test	Medium			~2		[30]
TuV	Suspension test	Medium			~2.2		[30]
FCV	Suspension test	Medium			>5.5		[30]
pH 12–12.5							
REO-3	Suspension test	Medium	3				[68]
Cox B	Suspension test	Medium	5				[69]
Echo 11	Suspension test	Medium	6				[68]
FMDV	Suspension test	Medium	>3.5				[39]
NaOH, 0.1 M (~pH 13)							
BVDV	Suspension test	Medium				2.5	[70]
HAV	Suspension test	Medium				2.7	[59]
SV40	Suspension test	Medium				3.9	[70]

Virus[a]	Method	Soil/Matrix[b]	Log_{10} Reduction after				References
			≤ 1 min	10 min	30 min	1 hr	
HAV	Stainless steel	5% serum		3.0			[43]
HAV	Stainless steel	90% plasma		3.6			[43]
CPV	Stainless steel	5% serum		3.5			[43]
CPV	Stainless steel	90% plasma		5.2			[43]
MVM	Suspension test	Medium	>4.7				[71]
MVM	Suspension test	Medium		>4			[66]
CPV	Suspension test	Medium				5.6	[70]
PV	Suspension test	Medium				5.9	[70]
AdV-2	Suspension test	Medium				>6.9	[70]
AdV-5	Suspension test	Medium		>6			[72]
NaOH, 0.5 M (~pH 13.7)							
HAV	suspension test	Medium				2.4	[59]
PV	suspension test	Medium				4.1	[63]
NaOH, 0.75 M (~pH 13.9)							
Avian Reo	Suspension test	Medium			4		[73]
PV	Suspension test	Medium			5.1		[73]
Bovine Rota	Suspension test	Medium			>6		[73]

[a]*See* ***Table 1*** *for abbreviations used for viruses.*
[b]*Medium, culture medium.*
Entries in purple font indicate results from undiluted or diluted formulations with microbicidal active ingredients.

Table 7.
Efficacy of high pH against non-enveloped viruses.

8. Inactivation of non-enveloped viruses by aldehydes

Aldehydes, such as glutaraldehyde, formaldehyde, and *ortho*-phthaldehyde, are widely used for sterilization, high-level disinfection for critical and semi-critical medical devices, biomanufacturing, and preservation. Their use for regular disinfection, sanitization, or antisepsis has been more limited, primarily due to human toxicity concerns. The efficacy of aldehydes, similar to the case for other types of actives, is concentration-dependent. There have been limited side-by-side comparison studies of the susceptibility of non-enveloped viruses to aldehydes; however, it may be concluded that animal parvoviruses seem to be less susceptible than other viruses, such as poliovirus, hepatitis A virus, feline calicivirus, adenovirus, reovirus, and rotavirus [74]. Within the parvoviruses, porcine parvovirus seems to be less susceptible to aldehydes than minute virus of mice (**Table 8**).

9. General order of susceptibility of non-enveloped viruses to chemical inactivation

In the simplified hierarchy of susceptibility of pathogens to microbicides concept, small non-enveloped viruses are considered less susceptible than large non-enveloped viruses, and both groups of non-enveloped viruses are believed to be less

Virus[a]	Method	Soil/Matrix[b]	Log_{10} Reduction after				References
			5 min	10 min	30 min	60 min	
Glutaraldehyde, 0.02%							
HAV	Suspension test	Medium			3.0		[75]
Glutaraldehyde, 0.05%							
MVM	Suspension test	Medium	0.5		1.5	2.8	[47]
MVM	Stainless steel	Medium	0.5		1.2	1.4	[47]
REO-3	Suspension test	Medium	3.3		>5		[47]
REO-3	Stainless steel	Medium	3.3		5.3		[47]
Glutaraldehyde, ~0.1%							
PPV	Stainless steel	BSA	1.7–2.8				[34]
MVM	Stainless steel	BSA	2.5–3.3				[34]
PV1	Suspension test	Medium			>3		[76]
FCV	Suspension test	Medium			5		[48]
AdV-5	Stainless steel	BSA	4.9–6.3				[34]
Rotavirus	Suspension test	Medium	>5				[56]
Glutaraldehyde, 2%							
PPV	Stainless steel	Erythrocytes + BSA		3.6			[26]
MVM	Stainless steel	Erythrocytes + BSA		>4.4			[26]
PV1	Glass	Medium	>4				[31]
Formaldehyde, 2%							
AdV-5	Suspension test	Medium				>5.0	[77]
Ortho-phthaldehyde, 0.55%							
PPV	Stainless steel	Erythrocytes + BSA		3.6			[26]
MVM	Stainless steel	Erythrocytes + BSA		>4.			[26]

*[a]See **Table 1** for abbreviations used for viruses.*
[b]BSA, bovine serum albumin; medium, culture medium; RT, room temperature.
Entries in purple font indicate results from original or diluted formulations with microbicidal active ingredients.

Table 8.
Efficacy of aldehydes against non-enveloped viruses.

susceptible than enveloped viruses. The hierarchy concept also assumes that the ranking applies to all types of microbicidal actives. Additionally, the hierarchy concept can generally lead to common notions that viruses that share similar virological properties (e.g., same family or genus of virus) may be expected to display similar degrees of susceptibility and that the smaller a virus is, the less susceptible it will be to microbicides in general.

These generalizations are correct, to a degree. For example, most enveloped viruses are indeed more susceptible than non-enveloped viruses to chemical inactivation. It should be noted though that exceptions to the hierarchy concept do exist, e.g., especially in the case of viral susceptibility to acids and alkalines [22], and exceptions are not uncommon for certain other chemistries. The hierarchy concept was never applied specifically to physical inactivation approaches, nor should it be. The evidence for heat inactivation, UV inactivation, and gamma irradiation indicates differing rankings of susceptibility to these modalities. Envelope status and particle size do not, in each case, relate to susceptibility for inactivation by these physical approaches [22, 78–80].

The validity of the hierarchy concept *among non-enveloped viruses* is much more blurred. Firstly, the order of susceptibility among non-enveloped viruses, if any generalization may be made, is dependent upon the type of chemistry, and there is no universal order that holds true for all types of chemistries. Secondly, large non-enveloped viruses (adenoviruses, reovirus, rotavirus, etc.) are *not* always more susceptible than small non-enveloped viruses (parvoviruses, picornaviruses, caliciviruses, etc.). Thirdly, viruses within the same group (e.g., same family or genus) can exhibit profound and unequivocal differences in susceptibility. Finally, the rankings between viruses can be flipped (reversed), or nonexistent, depending on the type of microbicide. This implies that caution should be taken when interpreting the hierarchy concept for making predictions of efficacy for the non-enveloped viruses.

The accuracy and usefulness of a hierarchy concept can be improved if the model is broken into separate chemistries for non-enveloped viruses, since many viruses do exhibit a reliable and consistent trend of susceptibility for a specific type of chemical. **Table 9** and **Figure 2** provide a summary of the relative order of susceptibility for selected non-enveloped viruses under specific types of chemistry.

Chemical	Lower susceptibility	Medium susceptibility	Higher susceptibility
Ethanol	Animal parvovirus	Poliovirus	Murine norovirus
	Simian virus 40	Foot and mouth disease virus	Rhinovirus
	Hepatitis A virus	Human norovirus	Adenovirus 5
	Enterovirus 71	Feline calicivirus	Rotavirus
		Adenovirus 2, 8	
Isopropanol	Animal parvovirus	Adenovirus 5, 8	Simian virus 40
	Hepatitis A virus	Murine norovirus	Rotavirus
	Enterovirus 71		
	Poliovirus		
	Feline calicivirus		
NaOCl	Porcine parvovirus	Minute virus of mice	Feline calicivirus
	Hepatitis A virus	Hepatitis A virus	Adenovirus
		Poliovirus	Rotavirus
		Enterovirus 71	
		Murine norovirus	
H_2O_2	Animal parvovirus	Poliovirus	Rhinovirus
	Hepatitis A virus	Murine norovirus	Feline calicivirus
		Adenovirus	Rotavirus
PAA	Animal parvovirus	Poliovirus	Feline calicivirus
	Hepatitis A virus		Murine norovirus
			Adenovirus
QAC	Animal parvovirus	Feline calicivirus	Rotavirus
	Poliovirus	Murine norovirus	Rhinovirus
	Adenovirus 8, 25	Adenovirus 5	Coxsackievirus A11

Chemical	Lower susceptibility	Medium susceptibility	Higher susceptibility
Low pH	Minute virus of mice	Human parvovirus 4	Feline calicivirus
	Hepatitis A virus		Rhinovirus
	Poliovirus		Foot and mouth disease virus
	Enterovirus 71		Enterovirus EV-D68
	Coxsackievirus A9		Human parvovirus B19
	Murine norovirus		
	Rotavirus		
	Reovirus		
High pH	Bovine viral diarrhea virus	Reovirus *(enveloped virus)*	Murine minute virus
		Simian virus 40	Feline calicivirus
		Hepatitis A virus	Adenovirus
		Canine parvovirus	Rotavirus
		Poliovirus	Foot and mouth disease virus
		Murine norovirus	
		Tulane virus	
Aldehydes	Porcine parvovirus	Minute virus of mice	Poliovirus
			Hepatitis A virus
			Feline calicivirus
			Adenovirus
			Reovirus
			Rotavirus

Abbreviations used: H_2O_2, hydrogen peroxide; NaOCl, sodium hypochlorite; PAA, peracetic acid; QAC, quaternary ammonium compound.

Table 9.
Relative order of susceptibility of non-enveloped viruses to chemical inactivation.

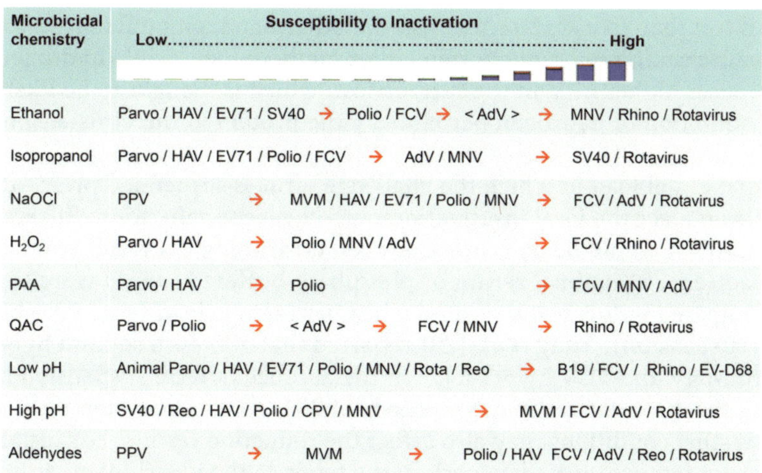

Figure 2.
Relative order of susceptibility of non-enveloped viruses per microbicidal chemistry. Note: various types of adenoviruses exhibit different degrees of susceptibility to ethanol and quaternary ammonium compounds.

10. Discussion

The Spaulding concept of the hierarchy of susceptibility of pathogens to microbicidal inactivation, along with its modifications, has been widely influential. Multiple industries as well as regulatory agencies have adopted or referenced this concept to various degrees [9, 10, 81, 82]. The concept does provide a good tool for understanding the innate differences and trending of susceptibility among various types of pathogens. For the most part, the hierarchy is insightful and valuable. It is particularly helpful when a pathogen is newly emerged, and limited or no knowledge is yet available regarding its level of susceptibility to microbicides [83, 84]. In fact, the United States Environmental Protection Agency (U.S. EPA) and Centers for Disease Control and Prevention (U.S. CDC) use the hierarchy concept as the basis of the Emerging Viral Pathogen Guidance for Antimicrobial Pesticides and public hygiene [10, 82, 85, 86] specifically to deal with just such a possibility.

It should be cautioned, however, that the hierarchy concept is largely oversimplified and by no means perfect [87]. For viruses, although enveloped viruses are usually more susceptible than non-enveloped viruses, certain enveloped viruses such as bovine viral diarrhea virus can be less susceptible than some non-enveloped viruses (e.g., feline calicivirus) under certain chemistries (e.g., low pH and high pH).

The accuracy and applicability of the hierarchy concept are more complex and limited among non-enveloped viruses. The trending is highly dependent on the type of chemistry; and the size of the virion is not always a primary determinant of viral susceptibility among non-enveloped viruses. If a clearer and more consistent trending can be identified among non-enveloped viruses, albeit only specific to a given type of chemistry, the knowledge should be useful.

To generalize an order of susceptibility, for a specific chemistry, data from side-by-side studies wherein viruses are evaluated concurrently by the same test method and under the same conditions should, ideally, be used. When results from different studies are used, caution should be taken to exclude conditional or case-specific differences that result from the test methodology and/or condition. For instance, a surface (carrier) test may give different $\log_{10}$ reduction results than a suspension test of the same microbicide or formulation under certain situations [88]. For example, the data of Kindermann et al. [47] and Tyler et al. [31] indicate that sodium hypochlorite causes a higher $\log_{10}$ reduction value (LRV) when tested in a suspension test than in a surface test. On the other hand, glutaraldehyde has been found to cause similar log reduction in either methodology, while hydrogen peroxide causes higher LRV in the surface test, which is thought to be likely related to the consumption of hydrogen peroxide by the protein in the virus-suspending solution [31].

The organic soil load in which the challenge virus is suspended prior to inoculation can also impact the viral inactivation outcome, especially for oxidizers, alcohols, and QAC. It would be inaccurate or even misleading if a result from a light organic load (e.g., 5% animal serum or phosphate-buffered saline) were to be directly compared with a test that used a heavier organic load (e.g., 90% blood or 20% fecal suspension). Tung *et al.* [29] reported that 500 ppm sodium hypochlorite inactivated MNV and FCV by ~3-$\log_{10}$ in the absence of fecal suspension but only 0–0.5 $\log_{10}$ for these viruses in the presence of 20% fecal suspension.

Other testing conditions may also affect the reduction results. For instance, a higher contact temperature may work in the favor of the virucide under investigation, which may result in a higher log reduction. Nemoto et al. [56] reported that a 0.125% glutaraldehyde solution completely inactivated rotavirus after 10 min under ambient temperature, but not when evaluated on ice. The pH and other components in the product formulation could also affect the viral reduction outcome, presumably by activating the chemical and/or by a synergistic or additive effect between the pH and the active chemical [22, 39, 89]. The efficacy of formulated versus non-formulated microbicides may differ even within the same type and concentration of active(s). For example, formulated QAC and ethanol products have been reported to exhibit strong activities against certain non-enveloped viruses albeit the efficacy may be weaker for non-formulated solutions [45, 54, 90, 91]. Therefore, the formulation of the microbicidal active must be considered. The viral stock (i.e., inoculum) preparation method and the challenge viral titer may also affect the reported viral reduction efficacy. For example, purified virus may be more susceptible than crude virus preparations [49]; viral clumps can make the virus less susceptible [92]; and a higher viral challenge titer could make the chemical harder to achieve an expected $\log_{10}$ reduction. Sometimes, viruses propagated in different host cell types may behave differently. It would therefore be ideal if all studies could use a standardized viral preparation and infectivity assay protocol. This is, of course, practically challenging. Last, but not least, the method for preparing the microbicide and the verification of the active concentration might also differ from lab to lab, thus potentially influencing the efficacy results obtained.

Despite these practically hard-to-avoid differences in test methodology and conditions, some generalizations on the pattern of susceptibility among non-enveloped viruses can still be made with confidence. For instance, it is quite apparent that the *Picornaviridae* family of viruses do not always exhibit a similar level of susceptibility to each other [16, 93]; and even the genus is not a good predictor for susceptibility to microbicides within this family. This reflects the ability of certain members of this family to infect the gastrointestinal tract (i.e., enteroviruses), while others infect primarily the respiratory system. The variation of susceptibility within this viral family is particularly striking for ethanol, hydrogen peroxide, QAC, and low pH.

The family *Caliciviridae* is another example of the existence of unequivocal intrafamily differences in susceptibility to microbicides [16]. For feline calicivirus and murine norovirus (the two most commonly used surrogate viruses for human norovirus), not only can their levels of susceptibility be very different, but the relative order of susceptibility between these two family members can be entirely reversed. For instance, murine norovirus is susceptible to ethanol but not very susceptible to low pH, whereas feline calicivirus is not very susceptible to ethanol but quite susceptible to low pH. For some other types of chemicals, such as peracetic acid and QAC, notable differences in susceptibility to these two viruses are not observed. Given the importance of human norovirus to public health and the lack of a convenient and robust tissue culture model for the virus, a more detailed research and discussion are needed with respect to the choice of feline calicivirus and murine norovirus as the best surrogate for evaluating inactivation products against human norovirus. This topic has been discussed extensively [94–96].

Different types of adenoviruses seem to exhibit varying degrees of susceptibility to ethanol and QAC. For example, adenovirus type 5 appears to be notably more susceptible to ethanol than are adenovirus types 2 and 8. In general, however, adenoviruses are more susceptible than many other non-enveloped viruses. Considering that adenovirus type 5 is listed as one of the allowable challenge viruses for a generic or "broad-spectrum" virucidal efficacy claim (i.e., a product that is effective for adenovirus type 5 may be considered effective against all viruses) [97, 98], this practice may not represent a challenge and lead to an insufficient safety margin, which is not supported by the published data.

Parvoviruses are among the smallest of non-enveloped viruses. The animal parvoviruses (e.g., minute virus of mice, porcine parvovirus, bovine parvovirus, canine parvovirus, etc.) are considered to exhibit very low susceptibility to chemical inactivation [99] and are commonly used as a worst-case model for viral inactivation studies. This literature review generally supports this notion, although it should be noted that the animal parvoviruses do not appear to represent a worst-case challenge for high-pH inactivation, and porcine parvovirus seems less susceptible than minute virus of mice at times. Additionally, human parvovirus B19 seems especially susceptible to acid treatment [100].

It has been observed that the particle size of a virus is not an exclusive or even a primary determinant of susceptibility to microbicides for non-enveloped viruses, albeit this characteristic may play a role. There are numerous reports demonstrating that larger non-enveloped viruses, such as adenoviruses and reoviruses, are less susceptible than some of the smaller non-enveloped viruses for certain chemistries. Interestingly though, rotavirus, a large non-enveloped virus, indeed seems to be the most susceptible among non-enveloped viruses, except to low pH.

The mechanisms underlying the large variation in susceptibility among non-enveloped viruses and the chemistry dependency are not always clear, but they could presumably be related to the physicochemical properties of the virus as well as the mechanisms of action of the chemical inactivants. For alcohols, for instance, it has been proposed that the hydrophobicity or hydrophilicity of the viral particles is an important determinant of susceptibility [101]. Poliovirus, which is hydrophilic, is more susceptible to ethanol than it is to isopropyl alcohol. This is attributed to the fact that ethanol is more hydrophilic than isopropanol. In comparison, the hydrophobic simian virus 40 is susceptible to isopropanol but not to ethanol [101]. Enterovirus 71 (EV71) and enterovirus EV-D68 (EV-D68) are both enteroviruses in the family *Picornaviridae*. Despite both infecting the gastrointestinal tract, EV71 displays low susceptibility to low pH, while EV-D68 is acid-labile. This can be explained by the observed acid-induced uncoating for EV-D68 but not for EV71 [67].

A review of the relative order of susceptibility for non-enveloped viruses under each chemistry reveals that the order for some chemicals (e.g. aldehydes) seems to fit the traditional hierarchy concept well (e.g., parvoviruses are less susceptible than larger viruses); but the order for some other chemistries (e.g., low pH) does not seem to agree with the concept as well.

The variability in viral susceptibility to physical treatments is not covered in this chapter; however, a marked degree of variation also exists for physical treatments, both within non-enveloped viruses and between enveloped and non-enveloped viruses [12, 16, 21, 49]. A comparison of the order of susceptibility of viruses to chemical versus physical treatments and an exploration of the underlying mechanisms would be interesting and revealing.

11. Conclusions

This chapter reviewed the literature on chemical inactivation of non-enveloped viruses, with an emphasis on the relative difference and trending of susceptibility among some relevant (from a public health perspective) non-enveloped viruses under each type of chemistry. The traditional concept of a hierarchy of susceptibility to microbicides provides a useful tool in understanding and predicting the susceptibility of a pathogen; however, the concept tends to be oversimplified. The order of susceptibility among non-enveloped viruses depends on the type of chemistry, and there is no universal order that holds true for all types of chemistries. Picornaviruses and caliciviruses exhibit a particularly high degree of intrafamily variation, and the order may even be reversed between viruses, depending on the chemistry. Additionally, larger non-enveloped viruses are not always more susceptible than some of the smaller non-enveloped viruses. It may be inappropriate to consider adenovirus type 5 as a worst-case non-enveloped virus; and even the animal parvoviruses, universally considered among the least susceptible to chemical inactivation, do not actually represent the least susceptible virus type for certain chemistries.

Acknowledgements

The author thanks Drs. Raymond Nims and M. Khalid Ijaz for the critical review of the manuscript and discussion.

Conflict of interest

The author declares no conflict of interest.

Author details

Sifang Steve Zhou
Microbac Laboratories, Inc., Sterling, Virginia, USA

*Address all correspondence to: steve.zhou@microbac.com

References

[1] Kampf G, Todt D, Pfaender S, Steinmann E. Persistence of coronaviruses on inanimate surfaces and their inactivation with biocidal agents. Journal of Hospital Infection. 2020; **104**(3):246-251

[2] Wiggins RC. Prion stability and infectivity in the environment. Neurochemical Results. 2009;**34**(1): 158-168

[3] Doetsch RN, Cook TM. Introduction to Bacteria and Their Ecobiology. Berlin: Springer Science & Business Media; 1973. ISBN 978-94-015-1137-7

[4] Spaulding EH. Chemical sterilization of surgical instruments. Surgical and Gynecological Observations. 1939;**69**: 738-744

[5] Spaulding EH. Chemical disinfection of medical and surgical materials. In: Lawrence CA, Block SS, editors. Disinfection, Sterilization, and Preservation. Philadelphia: Lea & Febiger; 1968. pp. 517-531

[6] Spaulding EH. Chemical disinfection and antisepsis in the hospital. Journal of Hospital Research. 1972;**9**:5-31

[7] Russell AD. Bacterial resistance to disinfectants: Present knowledge and future problems. Journal of Hospital Infection. 1998;**43**:S57-S68

[8] Sattar SA. Hierarchy of susceptibility of viruses to environmental surface disinfectants: A predictor of activity against new and emerging viral pathogens. Journal of the AOAC International. 2007;**90**(6):1655-1658

[9] U.S. EPA. Draft White Paper—Consideration of Disinfection Hierarchy Concepts in the Registration of Antimicrobial Products. Washington, USA: US Environmental Protection Agency; 2015

[10] U.S. CDC. Chemical disinfectants—guideline for disinfection and sterilization in healthcare facilities. Atlanta, USA:; U.S. Centers for Disease Control and Prevention; 2008

[11] Rutala WA, Weber DA, HICPAC. Guideline for Disinfection and Sterilization in Healthcare Facilities, 2008. (http://www.cdc.gov/hicpac/Disinfection_Sterilization/4_0efficacyDS.html#a2)

[12] Nims R, Plavsic M. Identification of worst-case model viruses for selected viral clearance steps. BioProcessing Journal. 2014;**13**:6-13

[13] Gelderblom HR. Structure and Classification of Viruses. in Medical Microbiology. 4th ed. Baron S, editor. Galveston: University of Texas Medical Branch at Galveston; 1996

[14] Fauquet CM. Taxonomy, classification and nomenclature of viruses. In: Granoff A, Webster RG, editors. Encyclopedia of Virology. Amsterdam, Ne therlands: Elsevier; 1999.1730–1756

[15] ICTV reports on virus taxonomy. https://talk.ictvonline.org/ictv-reports/

[16] Nims RW, Zhou SS. Intra-family differences in efficacy of inactivation of small non-enveloped viruses. Biologicals. 2016;**44**(5):456-462

[17] Alvarez ME, Brien RT. Mechanisms of inactivation of poliovirus by chlorine dioxide and iodine. Applied and Environmental Microbiology. 1982;**44**: 1064-1071

[18] Bieker JM. Chemical Inactivation of Viruses. Manhattan, Kansas: Kansas State University; 2006. http://hdl.handle.net/2097/226

[19] Biering H, Denzin S, von Rheinbaben F, Meyer B. Virucidal

Composition. Organization WIP, WO/2008/049454, editor. 2006.

[20] Lin Q, Lim JYC, Xue K, Yew PYM, Owh C, Chee PL, et al. Sanitizing agents for virus inactivation and disinfection. Viewpoints. 2020;**24**:e16

[21] Li JW, Xin ZT, Wang XW, Zheng JL, Chao FH. Mechanisms of inactivation of hepatitis a virus by chlorine. Applied and Environmental Microbiology. 2002;**68**(10):4951-4955

[22] Nims R, Zhou SS, Plavsic M. Identification of worst-case model viruses for low and high pH inactivation. Bioprocessing Journal. 2017;**16**(1):7-14

[23] Verbund für Angewandte Hygiene (VAH), EV, et al. As a Biocidal Active Substance, Ethanol is Indispensable for Hygienic Hand Disinfection. (Authorized translation). 29 October 2020, online available from. https://vah-online.de/en/. German original to be published in HygMed. 2020;45(11)

[24] Kampf G. Efficacy of ethanol against viruses in hand disinfection. Journal of Hospital Infection. 2018; **98**(4):331-338

[25] Edmonds S, McCormack R, Zhou SS, Macinga D, Fricker C. Hand hygiene regimens for the reduction of risk in foodservice environments. Journal of Food Protection. 2012;**75**(7): 1303-1309

[26] Eterpi M, McDonnell G, Thomas V. Disinfection efficacy against parvoviruses compared with reference viruses. Journal of Hospital Infection. 2009;**73**(1):64-70

[27] Chang SC, Li WC, Huang KY, Huang YC, Chiu CH, Chen CJ, et al. Efficacy of alcohols and alcohol-based hand disinfectants against human enterovirus 71. Journal of Hospital Infection. 2013;**83**(4):288-293

[28] Abad FX, Pintó RM, Bosch A. Disinfection of human enteric viruses on fomites. FEMS Microbiology Letters. 1997;**156**:107-111

[29] Tung G, Macinga D, Arbogast J, Jaykus LA. Efficacy of commonly used disinfectants for inactivation of human noroviruses and their surrogates. Journal of Food Protection. 2013;**76**(7): 1210-1217

[30] Cromeans T, Park GW, Costantini V, Lee D, Wang Q, Farkas T, et al. Comprehensive comparison of cultivable norovirus surrogates in response to different inactivation and disinfection treatments. Applied and Environmental Microbiology. 2014; **80**(18):5743-5751

[31] Tyler R, Ayliffe GAJ, Bradley C. Virucidal activity of disinfectants: Studies with the poliovirus. Journal of Hospital Infection. 1990;**15**:339-345

[32] Park GW, Barclay L, Macinga D, Charbonneau D, Pettigrew CA, Vinjé J. Comparative efficacy of seven hand sanitizers against murine norovirus, feline calicivirus, and GII.4 norovirus. Journal of Food Protection. 2010;**73**(12): 2232-2238

[33] Uzuner H, Karadenizli A, Er DK, Osmani A. Investigation of the efficacy of alcohol-based solutions on adenovirus serotypes 8, 19 and 37, common causes of epidemic keratoconjunctivitis, after an adenovirus outbreak in hospital. Journal of Hospital Infection. 2018; **100**(3):30-36

[34] Rabenau HF, Steinmann J, Rapp I, Schwebke I, Eggers M. Evaluation of a virucidal quantitative carrier test for surface disinfectants. PLoS One. 2014; **9**(1):1-10

[35] Wang Y-H, Wang X-L, Song J, Song Q-Q, Luo X-N, Xia D, et al. Inactivation of human rhinovirus due to heat, UV irradiation and chemical disinfectants.

Journal of Antivirals and Antiretrovirals. 2017;**9**(4):96-101

[36] van Engelenburg FA, Terpstra FG, Schuitemaker H, Moorer WR. The virucidal spectrum of a high concentration alcohol mixture. Journal of Hospital Infection. 2002;**51**:121-125

[37] von Rheinbaben F, Wolff MH. Handbuch der viruswirksamen Desinfektion. Berlin: Springer Verlag; 2002

[38] Kampf G, Grotheerc D, Steinmann J. Efficacy of three ethanol-based hand rubs against feline calicivirus, a surrogate virus for norovirus. Journal of Hospital Infection. 2005;**60**(2):144-149

[39] Harada Y, Lekcharoensuk P, Furuta T, Taniguchi T. Inactivation of foot-and-mouth disease virus by commercially available disinfectants and cleaners. Biocontrol Science. 2015; **20**(3):205-208

[40] Kramer A, Galabov AS, Sattar SA, Döhner L, Pivert A, Payan C, et al. Virucidal activity of a new hand disinfectant with reduced ethanol content: Comparison with other alcohol-based formulations. Journal of Hospital Infection. 2006;**62**(1):98-106

[41] Steinmann J, Becker B, Bischoff B, Magulski T, Steinmann J, Steinmann E. Virucidal activity of formulation I of the World Health Organization's alcohol-based handrubs: Impact of changes in key ingredient levels and test parameters. Antimicrobial Resistance and Infection Control. 2013;**2**:34. http://www.aricjournal.com/content/2/1/34

[42] Kurtz JB, Lee TW, Parsons AJ. The action of alcohols on rotavirus, astrovirus and enterovirus. Journal of Hospital Infection. 1980;**1**(4):321-325

[43] Terpstra FG, van den Blink AE, Bos LM, Boots AGC, Brinkhuis FHM, Gijsen E, et al. Resistance of surface-dried virus to common disinfection procedures. Journal of Hospital Infection. 2007;**66**:332-338

[44] Park GW, Sobsey MD. Simultaneous comparison of murine norovirus, feline calicivirus, coliphage MS2, and GII.4 norovirus to evaluate the efficacy of sodium hypochlorite against human norovirus on a fecally soiled stainless steel surface. Foodborne Pathogens and Disease. 2011;**8**(9): 1005-1010

[45] Sattar SA, Jacobsen H, Springthorpe VS, Cusack TM, Rubino JR. Chemical disinfection to interrupt transfer of rhinovirus type 14 from environmental surfaces to hands. Applied and Environmental Microbiology. 1993;**59**:1579-1585

[46] Kadurugamuwa JL, Shaheen E. Inactivation of human enterovirus 71 and coxsackie virus A16 and hand, foot, and mouth disease. American Journal of Infection Control. 2011;**39**(9):788-789

[47] Kindermann J, Karbiener M, Leydold SM, Knotzer S, Modrof J, Kreil TR. Virus disinfection for biotechnology applications: Different effectiveness on surface versus in suspension. Biologicals. 2020;**64**:1-9

[48] Poschetto LF, Ike A, Papp T, Mohn U, Böhm R, Marschang RE. Comparison of the sensitivities of noroviruses and feline calicivirus to chemical disinfection under field-like conditions. Applied and Environmental Microbiology. 2007;**73**(17):5494-5500

[49] Kiryanova EV, Panteleeva LG, Shirman GA. Inactivation of simian rotavirus SA 11 by hydrogen peroxide. Zentralblatt-fuer-Hygiene-und-Umweltmedizin. 1993;**194**(3):301-312

[50] Li D, Baert L, Jonghe MD, Van Coillie E, Ryckeboer J, Devlieghere F, et al. Inactivation of murine norovirus 1,

coliphage φX174, and Bacillus fragilis phage B40-8 on surfaces and fresh-cut iceberg lettuce by hydrogen peroxide and UV light. Applied and Environmental Microbiology. 2011; **77**(4):1399-1404

[51] Fraisse A, Temmam S, Deboosere N, Guillier L, Delobel A, Maris P, et al. Comparison of chlorine and peroxyacetic-based disinfectant to inactivate feline calicivirus, murine norovirus and hepatitis a virus on lettuce. International Journal of Food Microbiology. 2011;**151**(1):98-104

[52] Girard M, Mattison K, Fliss I, Jean J. Efficacy of oxidizing disinfectants at inactivating murine norovirus on ready-to-eat foods. International Journal of Food Microbiology. 2016;**219**:7-11

[53] Sansebastiano G, Zoni R, Bigliardi L, Ghirardi E, Losio N. Comparative study on HAV and poliovirus 2 inactivation cinetics with peracetic acid. Igiene e Sanita Pubblica. 2003;**59**(5):319-329

[54] Gerba CP. Quaternary ammonium biocides: Efficacy in application. Applied and Environmental Microbiology. 2015;**81**(2):464-469

[55] Maillard J-V et al. Does microbicide use in consumer products promote antimicrobial resistance? A critical review and recommendations for a cohesive approach to risk assessment. Microbial Drug Resistance. 2013;**19**(5): 344-354

[56] Nemoto M, Bannai H, Tsujimura K, Yamanaka T, Kondo T. Virucidal effect of commercially available disinfectants on equine group a rotavirus. Journal of Veterinary Medical Science. 2014;**76**(7): 1061-1063

[57] Romanowski EG, Yates KA, Shanks RM, Kowalski RP. Benzalkonium chloride demonstrates concentration-dependent antiviral activity against adenovirus in vitro. Journal of Ocular Pharmacology and Therapeutics. 2019;**35**:311-314

[58] Bauman PA, Lawrence LA, Biesert L, Dichtelmüller H, Fabbrizzi F, Gajardo R, et al. Critical factors influencing prion inactivation by sodium hydroxide. Vox Sanguinis. 2006;**91**(1):34-40

[59] Sofer G, Lister DC, Boose JA. Inactivation methods grouped by virus. BioPharm International. 2003;**6**:S37–S42

[60] Yang B, Wang H, Kaleas K, Butler M, Franklin J, Bill A, et al. Clearance of porcine circovirus and porcine parvovirus from porcine-derived pepsin by low pH inactivation and cation exchange chromatography. Biotechnology Progress. 2020;**36**(4): e2968

[61] Baylis SA, Tuke PW, Miyagawa E, Blümel J. Studies on the inactivation of human parvovirus 4. Transfusion. 2013; **53**(10 Pt 2):2585-2592

[62] Duizer E, Bijkerk P, Rockx B, De Groot A, Twisk F, Koopmans M. Inactivation of caliciviruses. Applied and Environmental Microbiology. 2004; **70**(8):4538-4543

[63] Roberts PL, Lloyd D. Virus inactivation by protein denaturants used in affinity chromatography. Biologicals. 2007;**35**:343-347

[64] Zhou S. unpublished data

[65] Newman JF, Rowlands DJ, Brown F. A physico-chemical sub-grouping of the mammalian picornaviruses. Journal of General Virology. 1973;**18**(2): 171-180

[66] Boschetti N, Wyss K, Mischler A, Hostettler T, Kempf C. Stability of minute virus of mice against temperature and sodium hydroxide. Biologicals. 2003;**31**(3):181-185

[67] Liu Y, Sheng J, van Vliet ALW, Buda G, van Kuppeveld FJM, Rossmann MG. Molecular basis for the acid-initiated uncoating of human enterovirus D68. Proceedings of the National Academy of Sciences (USA). 2018;**115**(52):E12209-E12217

[68] Drulak MW, Wallbank AM, Lebtag I. The effectiveness of six disinfectants in inactivation of reovirus 3. Microbios. 1984;**163**:31-38

[69] Drulak M, Wallbank AM, Lebtag I, Werboski L, Poffenroth L. The relative effectiveness of commonly used disinfectants in inactivation of coxsackievirus B5. Journal of Hygiene, Cambridge. 1978;**81**:389-397

[70] Application note: Use of sodium hydroxide for cleaning and sanitizing chromatography media and systems. Amersham Biosciences. 2001; 18-1124-57 AD

[71] Borovec S, Broumis C, Adcock W, Fang R, Uren E. Inactivation kinetics of model and relevant blood-borne viruses by treatment with sodium hydroxide and heat. Biologicals. 1998;**26**(3): 237-244

[72] Jannat R, Hsu D, Maheshwari G. Inactivation of adenovirus type 5 by caustics. Biotechnology Progress. 2005; **21**(2):446-450

[73] Maris P, Fresnel R. Activité de divers désinfectants sur sept virus non enveloppés. Annales de Recherches Vétérinaires. 1986;**17**:433-439

[74] Lukula L, Chiossone C, Fanuel S, Suchmann D, Nims R, Zhou SS. Inactivation and disinfection of porcine parvovirus on a nonporous surface. Journal of Microbial & Biochemical Technology. 2017;**9**(5):232-236

[75] Passagot J, Crance JM, Biziagos E, Laveran H, Agbalika F, Deloince R. Effect of glutaraldehyde on the antigenicity and infectivity of hepatitis a virus. Journal of Virological Methods. 1987;**16**(1–2):21-28

[76] Bailly JL, Chambon M, Peigue-Lafeuille H, Laveran H, De Champs C, Beytout D. Activity of glutaraldehyde at low concentrations (less than 2%) against poliovirus and its relevance to gastrointestinal endoscope disinfection procedures. Applied and Environmental Microbiology. 1991;**57**(4):1156-1160

[77] Möller L, Schünadel L, Nitsche A, Schwebke I, Hanisch M, Laue M. Evaluation of virus inactivation by formaldehyde to enhance biosafety of diagnostic electron microscopy. Viruses. 2015;7(2):666-679

[78] Nims RW, Plavsic M. Intra-family and inter-family comparisons for viral susceptibility to heat inactivation. Journal of Microbial and Biochemical Technology. 2013;**5**:136-141

[79] Zhou SS, Wilde C, Chen Z, Kapes T, Purgill J, Nims R, et al. Thermal inactivation of feline calicivirus and herpes simplex virus type 1: Side-By-Side Suspension and Carrier Studies. Integrative Journal of Veterinary Science. 2020;**4**(1):1–6. DOI: 10.31038/IJVB.2020411

[80] Zhou SS, Wilde C, Chen Z, Kapes T, Purgill J, Nims R, et al. Carrier and liquid heat inactivation of poliovirus and adenovirus. In: Disinfection. London: IntechOpen; 2018. ISBN 978-953-51-6084-7

[81] Lin CS, Fuller J, Mayhall ES. Federal regulation of liquid chemical germicides by the U.S. Food and Drug Administration. In: Block S, editor. Disinfection, Sterilization, and Preservation. 5th ed. Philadelphia: Lippencott, Williams and Wilkens. 2001. pp. 881–917

[82] U.S. Environmental Protection Agency. Guidance to Registrants:

Process for Making Claims against Emerging Viral Pathogens not on EPA-registered Disinfectant Labels. 2016. https://www.epa.gov/sites/default/files/2016-09/documents/emerging_viral_pathogen_program_guidance_final_8_19_16_001_0.pdf

[83] Ijaz MK, Nims RW, Cutts TA, McKinney J, Gerba CP. Predicted and measured virucidal efficacy of microbicides for emerging/and re-emerging viruses associated with WHO priority diseases. In: Disinfection of Viruses. London: InTech Open; in press

[84] Ijaz MK, Sattar SA, Rubino JR, Nims RW, Gerba CP. Combating SARS-CoV-2: Leveraging microbicidal experiences with other emerging/re-emerging viruses. PeerJ. 2020;**8**:e9914. DOI: 10.7717/peerj.9914

[85] U.S. Environmental Protection Agency. Emerging Viral Pathogen Guidance for Antimicrobial Pesticides. https://www.epa.gov/pesticide-registration/emerging-viral-pathogen-guidance-antimicrobial-pesticides. 2021

[86] U.S. EPA, Final Summary of the Disinfection Hierarchy Workshop. US Environmental Protection Agency. USA: Washington; 2016

[87] Disinfection: Is it time to reconsider Spaulding? Journal of Hospital Infection. 2011;**78**:163-170

[88] Ijaz MK, Rubino JR. Should test methods for disinfectants use vertebrate virus dried on carriers to advance virucidal claims? Infection Control and Hospital Epidemiology. 2008;**29**(2):192-194

[89] Vaughn JM, Chen YS, et al. Inactivation of human and simian rotaviruses by chlorine. Applied and Environmental Microbiology. 1986; **51**(2):391-394

[90] Sattar SA, Jacobsen H, Rahman H, Cusack TM, Rubino JR. Interruption of rotavirus spread through chemical disinfection. Infection Control and Hospital Epidemiology. 1994;**15**(12): 751-756

[91] Macinga DR, Sattar SA, Jaykus L-A, Arbogast JW. Improved inactivation of nonenveloped enteric viruses and their surrogates by a novel alcohol-based hand sanitizer. Applied and Environmental Microbiology. 2008; **74**(16):5047-5052

[92] Gerba CP, Betancourt WQ. Viral aggregation: Impact on virus behavior in the environment. Environmental Science & Technology. 2017;**51**(13): 7318-7325

[93] Su Y, Han J, Li J, Ren Z, Huang L, Xu B, et al. Resistance of poliovirus 1 and enterovirus A71 against alcohol and other disinfectants. Journal of Virological Methods. 2021;**298**:114292. DOI: 10.1016/j.jviromet.2021.114292

[94] Nims R, Plavsic M. Inactivation of caliciviruses. Pharmaceuticals. 2013;**6**: 358-392

[95] Cannon JL, Papafragkou E, Park GW, Osborne J, Jaykus LA, Vinjé J. Surrogates for the study of norovirus stability and inactivation in the environment: A comparison of murine norovirus and feline calicivirus. Journal of Food Protection. 2006;**69**(11): 2761-2765

[96] Hoelzer K, Fanaselle W, Pouillot R, Van Doren JM, Dennis S. Virus inactivation on hard surfaces or in suspension by chemical disinfectants: Systematic review and meta-analysis of norovirus surrogates. Journal of Food Protection. 2013;**76**(6):1006-1016

[97] Health Canada. Guidance document—Safety and Efficacy Requirements for Hard Surface Disinfectant Drugs. 2014. https://www.canada.ca/en/health-canada/services/drugs-health-products/drug-products/

applications-submissions/guidance-documents/disinfectants/safety-efficacy-requirements-hard-surface-disinfectant-drugs.html

[98] EN 14476:2013+A2:2019(E). Chemical disinfectants and antiseptics—Quantitative suspension test for the evaluation of virucidal activity in the medical area—Test method and requirements (Phase 2/Step 1). European Standard, July 2019.

[99] United States Pharmacopeia <1050.1>. Design, evaluation, and characterization of viral clearance procedures

[100] Boschetti N, Niederhauser I, Kempf C, Stühler A, Löwer J, Blümel J. Different susceptibility of B19 virus and mice minute virus to low pH treatment. Transfusion. 2004;**44**(7):1079-1086

[101] Ionidis G, Hübscher J, Jack T, Becker B, Bischoff B, Todt D, et al. Development and virucidal activity of a novel alcohol-based hand disinfectant supplemented with urea and citric acid. BMC Infectious Diseases. 2016;**16**:77. DOI: 10.1186/s12879-016-1410-9

Section 2

Physical Inactivation Approaches

Chapter 7

Physical Inactivation of SARS-CoV-2 and Other Coronaviruses: A Review

Raymond W. Nims and Mark Plavsic

Abstract

Severe acute respiratory syndrome coronavirus 2 (SARS-CoV-2) is the virus responsible for the ongoing pandemic of Coronavirus Disease 2019 (COVID-19). Other members of the enveloped RNA virus family *Coronaviridae* have been responsible for a variety of human diseases and economically important animal diseases. Disinfection of air, environmental surfaces, and solutions is part of infection prevention and control (IPAC) for such viruses and their associated diseases. This article reviews the literature on physical inactivation (disinfection) approaches for SARS-CoV-2 and other coronaviruses. Data for thermal (heat) inactivation, gamma irradiation, and ultraviolet light in the C range (UVC) irradiation have been reviewed. As expected, the susceptibilities of different members of the *Coronaviridae* to these physical inactivation approaches are similar. This implies that knowledge gained for SARS-CoV-2 should be applicable also to its emerging mutational variants and to other future emerging coronaviruses. The information is applicable to a variety of disinfection applications, including IPAC, inactivation of live virus for vaccine or laboratory analytical use, and waste stream disinfection.

Keywords: coronaviruses, *D* value, gamma irradiation, SARS-CoV-2, thermal (heat) inactivation, UVC inactivation

1. Introduction

The ongoing pandemic of severe acute respiratory syndrome coronavirus 2 (SARS-CoV-2) and its associated disease, Coronavirus Disease 2019 (COVID-19), have resulted in the generation of a tremendous amount of literature on various aspects of the disease and the virus. Of importance to this chapter is the literature on physical disinfection strategies for the virus, and infection prevention and control (IPAC) strategies for reducing potential transmission of the virus. In addition, physical inactivation approaches are used for rendering patient samples safe for handling in laboratories conducting diagnostic assays. Certain physical inactivation approaches also are used as barrier technologies for rendering human and animal raw materials safe for use in biologics manufacture. The literature specific to SARS-CoV-2 that has been published in the past 18 months is supplemented by previous literature on other relevant human and animal coronaviruses. These include human coronavirus 229E (HCoV-229E), severe acute respiratory syndrome coronavirus (SARS-CoV), Middle East respiratory syndrome coronavirus (MERS-CoV), porcine epidemic diarrhea virus (PEDV), transmissible gastroenteritis virus (TGEV), porcine hemagglutinating encephalomyelitis virus (PHEV), and canine, feline, and bovine coronaviruses (this list is not all-inclusive). For the present review chapter, the authors searched the literature for gamma irradiation, electron beam, high pressure, UVC, and heat (thermal) inactivation of coronaviruses in general, and in particular, the specific coronaviruses listed above. No limits were placed on date of publication, although, for obvious reasons, the data on SARS-CoV-2 were obtained from papers published since 2019.

Strategies for IPAC of SARS-CoV-2 include an impressive arsenal of pharmaceutical (vaccines, palliative therapies) and non-pharmaceutical interventions (face mask usage, social distancing, testing, contact tracing and quarantine), as well as chemical and physical approaches for liquid, surface, and air disinfection and for personal hygiene. In this chapter, we have attempted to review the physical inactivation efficacy data for SARS-CoV-2 and other coronaviruses. Our primary emphasis in this review is on IPAC, but other applications of physical inactivation approaches, such as rendering laboratory samples safe for handling within a biosafety I or II facility, and barrier treatments for inactivating potential contaminants in biologics animal-derived materials, are discussed.

2. Overview of physical viral inactivation approaches

The most commonly employed physical approaches for inactivating viruses are thermal (heat) inactivation (applied either to viruses in solutions or dried on surfaces); irradiation (applied to viruses in solutions, in solids, or dried on surfaces); and high pressure (most often employed for disinfection of food items). The irradiation approaches include gamma irradiation, X-irradiation, electron beam irradiation, and 254 nm ultraviolet light (UVC) irradiation. Irradiation with ultraviolet light in the A range and with visible light typically requires the addition of a photoactive chemical and, therefore, these are not truly physical approaches, but rather mixed physical/chemical approaches. The latter will not be dealt with in this chapter. Electron beam irradiation and high-pressure treatment are most commonly used for food preservation and the efficacy data to be found in the literature necessarily involve viruses of food concern (e.g., caliciviruses, astroviruses, reoviruses, picornaviruses, and adenoviruses) [1, 2]. Coronaviruses are not considered viruses of food concern [3] and, therefore, there are little or no data for inactivation of coronaviruses by electron beam irradiation and high-pressure treatment. As a result, there will be little discussion of these approaches in this chapter.

Physical inactivation approaches display efficacy for a broad range of viruses, including both lipid-enveloped and non-enveloped viruses. The factors determining virucidal efficacy for one virus type over another differ among the physical approaches. For instance, particle size appears to be the major determinant for inactivation efficacy of gamma, X-ray, and electron beam irradiation [4], while genomic structure (single vs. double strand, circularity, and relative content of pyrimidine dinucleotides) appears to be more important for determining UVC inactivation efficacy [5]. Thermal inactivation appears to be effective for both lipid-enveloped and non-enveloped viruses, and particle size does not appear to correlate with efficacy [6]. Having said this, the most highly resistant of viruses to heat inactivation are the non-enveloped parvoviruses, circoviruses, and polyomaviruses [6]. The orthogonality of mechanism of inactivation displayed by these physical approaches is convenient. If one approach is not practical for a given virus family, another approach may be applied. A good example is the parvovirus family of small non-enveloped viruses. These typically are highly resistant to thermal inactivation and to gamma, X-ray, and electron beam irradiation but are quite susceptible to UVC irradiation [7].

Physical inactivation approaches also differ with respect to the types of sample matrices that may be treated. Thermal inactivation has the broadest range of matrix types, including liquids and surfaces. Of course, temperatures high enough to inactivate viruses may have adverse impacts on the sample matrices being irradiated. Gamma radiation has high penetrability, and can be used for liquids and solids, though the matrix to be irradiated must be brought in close contact with a gamma source, and such sources are available only at specialized irradiation facilities. In order to minimize potential side effects of gamma irradiation (free radicals, heat) and to maintain the integrity of the sample matrix (such as bovine serum), the typical gamma irradiation process requires keeping the sample to be irradiated at very cold temperature (typically, such samples are kept on dry ice during irradiation) [8]. Electron beam radiation has low penetrability, so is typically used for thin items such as food items [1]. Due to its low penetrability, ultraviolet light irradiation is effective only if the radiation reaches all portions of the matrix being irradiated [9]. It is a line-of-sight approach. It is used for inactivating viruses on non-porous surfaces and liquids which have low UVC-absorbance characteristics [9].

An advantage of physical inactivation approaches is the first-order behavior typically displayed for inactivation of viruses (see **Box 1**). This enables one to make informed predictions of inactivation efficacy at temperatures, times, fluences that have not specifically been tested empirically.

First-order viral inactivation by physical approaches. One commonality among the physical inactivation approaches is that, as a generality, the $\log_{10}$ reduction in virus titer observed following treatment is first-order (linear) with respect to time in the case of heat inactivation, or with applied dose (fluence) in the case of irradiation. Of course, there are exceptions, which are sometimes attributed to mixed virus populations with differential susceptibility to the inactivation approach. It is likely that the biphasic or non-linear behavior attributed to such mixed populations is due to experimental artifact, including the inclusion of data points which approach the limit of detection of the titration assays used, or simply the fact that most of the available virus has already been inactivated. The typical first-order behavior of the physical inactivation approaches enables the calculation of decimal reduction values (*D*) for a given virus, corresponding to the thermal treatment time or irradiation fluence associated with a 1-$\log_{10}$ reduction in virus titer. Knowing such a *D* value allows one to adjust the thermal contact time or the irradiation fluence such that a desired $\log_{10}$ reduction value may be achieved for a given virus. For instance, in the tables to follow in this chapter, thermal inactivation *D* values are plotted against temperature to allow estimation of log reduction at any given time and temperature. Similarly, gamma irradiation and UVC irradiation efficacy are expressed in terms of $\log_{10}$ reduction per kGy (gamma irradiation) or $\log_{10}$ reduction per mJ/cm^2 fluence (UVC). This enables one to estimate the effectiveness of the irradiation approach for inactivating a given virus under conditions not tested empirically.

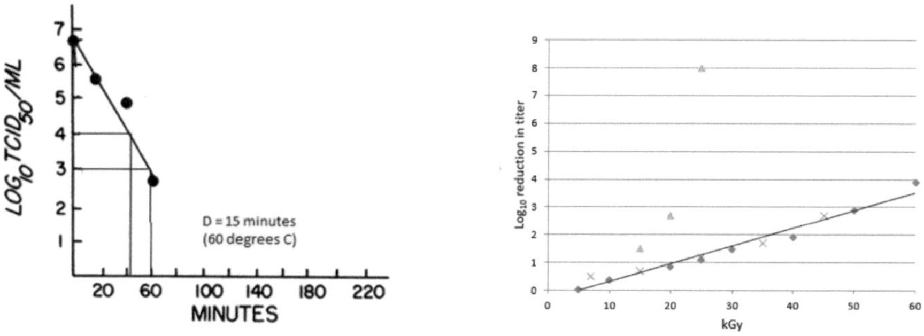

Box 1.
Left panel: calculation of a D value for heat inactivation of a parvovirus at 60 °C (from [10]); right panel, first-order behavior for two data sets (× and ◊) and one data set displaying non-linear behavior (△) for inactivation of a parvovirus by gamma irradiation (from [4]).

3. Inactivation of coronaviruses by gamma irradiation

Gamma irradiation is commonly used for sterilization of plasticware (especially tissue culture flasks, bottles, pipette tips, and pipettes). For such applications, a high fluence (hundreds of kGy) may be used to kill any prokaryotic microbes and viruses [11]. When it comes to disinfecting surfaces, again, sufficiently high fluences may be employed to kill any microbes and viruses. For disinfection of frozen or liquid solutions, care must be taken to balance the need for adequate sterilization with maintenance of the expected performance of the solutions being irradiated [4]. Gamma radiation interacts with solutions in different manners, depending on a number of factors, including the temperature of the solution and the presence of radiation-scavenging compounds. At very low temperatures (< −60°C, for instance, and in the presence of radiation scavengers, such as concentrated proteins), the radiation impacts on the solution itself are limited, and the impacts on suspended microbes are more selectively targeted to vital macromolecules such as genomic material. These effects are termed "direct" radiation effects. At temperatures above freezing and in the absence of scavenging compounds, effects termed "indirect" are imparted to the solution. These are characterized as radiolysis products attributed to the interaction of photons with water, forming oxygen radicals that can damage not only suspended microbes but also any biological materials in solutions. As a result of the above, inactivation of viruses in solutions, such as animal serum or culture medium containing serum, is typically accomplished by irradiating the sample matrices frozen on dry ice [4, 8].

As mentioned already, gamma radiation is highly penetrating, therefore is ideal for pathogen reduction in deeply frozen containers of animal serum and other biological samples. The data pertaining to efficacy of gamma irradiation for inactivating coronaviruses [12–16] are displayed in **Table 1**. These data were collected using deeply frozen tissue culture medium containing small amounts of bovine serum (i.e., the harvest medium containing the virus that comprised the viral stocks tested). In each case, the sample temperature during irradiation was maintained through use of dry ice, so that primarily the direct effects of the radiation on the viral macromolecules were to be expected. As expected, based on the known mechanism of action of gamma radiation on the viruses, and the relatively large particle size (60–136 nm) of the coronaviruses, the inactivating efficacies of gamma irradiation on SARS-CoV, MERS-CoV, and SARS-CoV-2 were similar in the reported studies [12–16]. The consensus data indicate an efficacy of 0.5–0.9 $\log_{10}$ inactivation per kGy of gamma radiation. At the typical range of fluences administered to frozen animal serum (25–45 kGy), as an example, one would therefore expect >12 $\log_{10}$ inactivation of coronaviruses (i.e., 0.5 $\log_{10}$ inactivation per kGy × 25 kGy). It may be predicted that

Virus[a]	**Temperature (°C)**	**Inactivation matrix**	***D* value (kGy)**	**Efficacy ($\log_{10}$/kGy)**	**Efficacy at 25 kGy ($\log_{10}$)**	**Ref.**
SARS-CoV-2	−80 (dry ice)	Culture medium	1.6	0.63	16	[12]
SARS-CoV-2	−80 (dry ice)	Culture medium	1.1	0.92	23	[13]
SARS-CoV	−80 (dry ice)	Culture medium	≤1.7	≤0.60	≤15	[14]
SARS-CoV	−80 (dry ice)	Culture medium	>0.15	ND[b]	ND	[15]
MERS-CoV	−80 (dry ice)	Culture medium	2.0	0.50	12	[16]

[a]*MERS-CoV, Middle East respiratory syndrome coronavirus; SARS-CoV-2, severe acute respiratory syndrome coronavirus 2; SARS-CoV, severe acute respiratory syndrome coronavirus.*
[b]*ND, not determined. The highest fluence tested (0.15 kGy) failed to cause ≥ one $\log_{10}$ inactivation.*

Table 1.
Efficacy of gamma irradiation for inactivating coronaviruses.

members of the coronavirus family, including future emerging species, should each be highly susceptible to inactivation by gamma radiation.

Greater efficacy for inactivating coronaviruses may be expected when irradiating solutions at higher temperatures (especially above freezing) and in the absence of radiation scavengers. This is due to the additional contribution of the indirect effects of gamma radiation. Of course, under these conditions, the matrix being irradiated may be degraded to the point where it no longer is useful for the intended application.

As indicated in the above, gamma irradiation should be considered a very effective physical approach for inactivating coronaviruses, such as SARS-CoV-2. Reports have suggested, for instance, the suitability of gamma irradiation for inactivation of SARS-CoV-2, while preventing loss of antigenic content, for use in preparing vaccines [17]. In a practical sense, however, the requirement for a gamma radiation source such as cobalt^{60} limit the general availability of this approach for routine use. Items or solutions to be gamma irradiated must be shipped to an irradiation facility to accomplish this.

4. Inactivation by UVC irradiation

As mentioned above, photons of light from various regions of the electromagnetic spectrum (i.e., visible, UVA, UVB, and UVC) have been used for inactivation of viruses. Available scientific literature indicates that light in the UVC range has the greatest efficacy for inactivating viruses, through a purely physical mechanism of action that does not depend on chemical radiation-sensitizing compounds. While visible light (405 nm) in the absence of photosensitizing agents has been shown to have efficacy for inactivating SARS-CoV-2, this activity is relatively weak, compared to that of UVC. For instance, a fluence of 288 mJ/cm^2 was required to cause a 2.58 $\log_{10}$ inactivation [18], equating to about 0.0090 $\log_{10}$/(mJ/cm^2), an order of magnitude greater than the UVC fluence required (see below). The reason for the unique efficacy of UVC light in the absence of sensitizing agents is thought to be the correspondence of the UVC light wavelength, typically 254 nm light from mercury vapor lamps, with the absorbance peaks of the target nucleic acids (~265 nm) [9, 19].

Only the efficacy of UVC light is discussed in the tables below. Unlike gamma irradiation, which can penetrate solids, UVC irradiation is a line-of-sight approach, which depends on exposure of target organisms to the radiation. The impacts to the target organism depend on the absorbed dose. As with gamma irradiation, the dose of UVC light applied can be expressed in a single fluence term that takes into account both dose rate and time. A variety of units have been used in the literature, which can lead to confusion when attempting to compare results between labs. We use the units mJ/cm^2 in this chapter, since most of the virus inactivation results to be found in the literature have been expressed in these units. Conversion of other fluence units, such as J/m^2 to mJ/cm^2 is straightforward, while exposures expressed in units of mW/cm^2 must be multiplied by the exposure time (in seconds) to convert to mJ/cm^2.

The mechanism of inactivation of viruses by UVC radiation is thought to involve interaction of the energetic photons with nucleic acids comprising the viral genome. Pyrimidine nucleotides (uracil, thymine, cytosine) are especially susceptible to the formation of covalent dimers following exposure to UVC. A more thorough discussion of mechanisms and pyrimidine dimer formation, and relevance for predicting efficacy for viruses of different genomic structure, is beyond the scope of this chapter. Readers are referred to excellent source papers [5, 20, 21].

There is some literature on coronavirus inactivation in liquid matrices by UVC radiation, and rather scanty information on irradiation of these viruses on solid surfaces or in aerosols. A summary of the evaluation of UVC efficacy for inactivating SARS-CoV-2 and other coronaviruses in liquid matrices is displayed in

Table 2. No attempt to cherry-pick the efficacy data has been made in assembling this table, although it will be readily apparent on review of this table that discrepant results in terms of *D* value and $\log_{10}$ inactivation per mJ/cm^2 have been reported. For an informed analysis of possible factors underlying these discrepant values, relating primarily to optical density of the liquid matrices and dosimetry difficulties, the reader is referred to Boegel et al. [19].

Neglecting the clearly discrepant values in this table, certain of which unfortunately have caused some confusion on the sensitivity of coronaviruses to UVC radiation [33], a consensus *D* value in the range of 0.5–2 mJ/cm^2 may be inferred. This *D* range corresponds to a consensus efficacy of 0.5–2 $\log_{10}$/mJ/cm^2 (**Table 2**). To put these *D* values into perspective, the most UVC-resistant viruses (adenoviruses and polyomaviruses), have UVC *D* values >50 mJ/cm^2 [6].

A summary of the evaluation of the inactivation of coronaviruses by UVC radiation on solid surfaces and in aerosols is provided in **Table 3**. As mentioned above, there are fewer reports for this topic within the literature. On a theoretical basis, UVC radiation accessibility to viruses dried on surfaces or present in aerosols should be optimal, therefore such considerations as impact of stirring or impact of matrix absorption of the radiation should not confound the efficacy results to the extent that these do in liquid matrix studies. Although the dataset in **Table 3** is limited, the agreement between observed *D* values between reports and between coronaviruses is fairly close, perhaps in keeping with the lessened impact of confounding factors mentioned above. The *D* values shown in **Table 3** also are in good agreement with the consensus *D* values (0.5–2 mJ/cm^2) from the liquid matrix studies.

Virus[a]	Wavelength (nm)	Inactivation matrix	*D* value (mJ/cm^2)	Efficacy ($\log_{10}$/mJ/cm^2)	Reference
SARS-CoV-2	254	Culture medium	1.7	0.59	[19]
SARS-CoV-2	254	Culture medium	6.7	0.15	[22]
SARS-CoV-2	254	Culture medium	1.8	0.56	[23]
SARS-CoV-2	254	Culture medium	0.5–7.5	0.13–2.0	[24]
SARS-CoV-2	282	Culture medium	12.5	0.080	[25]
SARS-CoV-2	254	Culture medium	98	0.010	[26]
SARS-CoV-2	265	Culture medium	0.6	1.7	[27]
SARS-CoV-2	254	Culture medium	0.016	Not calculated[b]	[28]
SARS-CoV	254	Culture medium	22	0.044	[29]
SARS-CoV	254	Culture medium	300	0.20	[15]
SARS-CoV	260	Culture medium	300	0.20	[30]
HCoV 229E	254	Culture medium	1.8	0.56	[19]
HCoV 229E	254	Culture medium	1.7	0.59	[31]
HCoV OC43	254	Culture medium	1.7	0.59	[19]
HCoV OC43	267	PBS	2	0.5	[32]
MHV	254	Culture medium	1.2	0.82	[19]
MHV	254	Culture medium	1.1	0.91	[31]

[a]HCoV, human coronavirus; MHV, mouse hepatitis virus; PBS, phosphate buffered saline. SARS-CoV, severe acute respiratory syndrome coronavirus; SARS-CoV-2, severe acute respiratory syndrome coronavirus 2.
[b]The reported inactivation kinetics were not first-order.

Table 2.
Efficacy of Ultraviolet C (UVC) irradiation for inactivating coronaviruses in liquid matrices.

Virus[a]	Wavelength (nm)	Surface/Aerosol	*D* value (mJ/cm^2)	Efficacy ($log_{10}/mJ/cm^2$)	Reference
SARS-CoV-2	254	Plastic	1.4	0.71	[23]
SARS-CoV-2	222	Plastic	1.2	0.83	[34]
SARS-CoV-2	260–285	Stainless steel	1.6	0.63	[35]
SARS-CoV-2	260–285	N95 mask fabric	21	0.05	[35]
HCoV 229E	222	Aerosol	0.56	1.8	[36]
HCoV OC43	222	Aerosol	0.39	2.6	[36]
MHV	254	Aerosol	0.66	1.5	[37]
IBV	254	Aerosol	13.8	0.07	[38]

[a]*HCoV, human coronavirus; IBV, infectious bronchitis virus; MHV, mouse hepatitis virus; SARS-CoV-2, severe acute respiratory syndrome coronavirus 2*

Table 3.
Efficacy of Ultraviolet C (UVC) irradiation for inactivating coronaviruses on surfaces or in aerosols.

For general reviews of UVC inactivation of coronaviruses in various matrices, the reader may also consult Boegel et al. [19], Hadi et al. [20], Chiappa et al. [39], and Helßling et al. [40]. Pendyala et al. [21] used efficacy modeling based on pyrimidine dinucleotide content to predict UVC efficacy for inactivating various alpha-, beta-, and gamma-coronaviruses. The conclusion of the modeling was that coronaviruses, as a family, are highly susceptible to UVC, and the *D* values obtained in the modeling for the various coronaviruses ranged from 18.0 to 28.1 J/m^2 (1.8–2.8 mJ/cm^2), aligning well with the consensus *D* values from **Tables 2** and **3**.

The data presented suggest that UVC irradiation is a very effective physical approach for inactivating coronaviruses, such as SARS-CoV-2. It is not surprising, therefore, that UVC has been proposed for a variety of applications, including indoor air sanitization [36, 41–44], inactivation of coronaviruses in water [33] or other solutions, inactivation of biological samples for downstream use in assays [22], and surface hygiene [34, 45], including sanitization of personal protective equipment [35, 46, 47].

5. Thermal (heat) inactivation

As is the case for gamma irradiation, heat can be highly penetrating, depending upon the inactivation matrix. For instance, heat transfer within liquids is typically efficient, so heat inactivation is a commonly employed method for inactivating adventitious agents (including viruses) in solutions. Heat inactivation is also commonly utilized for decontaminating non-porous surfaces. For some time, there has existed a dogma that heat inactivation of viruses is more effective when applied to solutions (liquid or wet inactivation) than to surfaces (carrier or dry inactivation). Exceptions to this have been noted recently [48, 49], and it is more correct to state that relative efficacy for wet vs. dry heating may depend upon the specific virus being inactivated.

The mechanisms underlying inactivation of viruses by heat are thought to be the same for both enveloped and non-enveloped viruses. The treatment is thought to result in leaky protein capsids, which allow penetration of the capsid by nucleases and loss of capsid contents to the environment. In either case, nucleases would be expected to rapidly degrade the genomic material and render the viruses non-infectious [50]. If this mechanism is correct, heat inactivation efficacy should be similar for enveloped and non-enveloped viruses. Indeed, examination of wet heat inactivation data across virus families confirms this conclusion [6]. While certain viruses (e.g., animal parvoviruses and polyomaviruses) exhibit unusually high heat resistance, in general non-enveloped viruses do not appear to be significantly more resistant to heat than enveloped viruses [6].

The literature on heat inactivation of coronaviruses, including SARS-CoV-2, is extensive. The reports generally contain information on efficacy of one or more temperatures evaluated for one or more time periods. These studies [15, 29, 30, 51–65] generally do not report *D* values, only $\log_{10}$ reduction in titer obtained from heating at a given temperature for set time periods (e.g., 56°C for 30 min). Examples of this sort of heat inactivation data are given in **Table 4**. Note that in **Table 4**, data for temperatures greater than 45°C are displayed. Results at lower temperatures are associated with a great deal of variability. For readers interested in coronavirus stability at the lower temperatures (ambient to ~45°C), the following review papers may be consulted [65–70]. The data in **Table 4** indicate that inactivation of coronaviruses at temperatures between 48 and 54°C may be incomplete at exposure times up to 60 min. Temperatures ≥56°C are generally quite effective at exposure times of 10 min or greater, while temperatures ≥80°C are very effective within 1 or 2 min of exposure. Similar efficacies of heat inactivation for various members of the *Coronaviridae* are observed.

Relatively few reports of heat inactivation on carriers (dry heat) have been published for coronaviruses (**Table 5**). These studies [35, 71–73] have been concerned primarily with decontamination of personal protective equipment (gowns, N95 respirators) for reuse, although Fischer et al. [35] and Biryukov et al. [72] also evaluated inactivation of SARS-CoV-2 on stainless steel carriers. Estimates of *D* values for heat inactivation on surfaces (**Table 5**) range from ~7 min at 60°C (PEDV) to 11–35 min at 55–70°C (SARS-CoV-2).

The most useful heat inactivation results are expressed in terms of *D* values measured at three or more temperatures. The latter datasets enable the plotting of *D* vs. temperature curves, which, in turn, enable comparison of the efficacy of the heat inactivation results obtained in different laboratories, as well as estimation of *D* at non-measured temperatures. It should be noted that, while the kinetics of inactivation of viruses by heat at a given temperature are expected to be first-order with respect to time, the relationship between *D* and temperature is more complex [74]. In the past, the latter relationship has been plotted on semi-log scales ($\log_{10} D$ vs. time), resulting in linear plots from which *Z* values (°C per $\log_{10}$ change in *D*) could be calculated. These *Z* values could then be used to estimate *D* at non-measured temperatures. More recently, it has been discovered that the plot of *D* vs. temperature can be fit accurately with the power function. Examples of such plots for coronavirus heat inactivation are shown in **Figures 1** and **2**. The resulting line equation coefficients (**Table 6**) then may be used, in a more intuitive and straightforward manner, to estimate *D* at non-measured temperatures [74].

Some authors [66, 75] have taken the interesting and informative approach of combining the heat inactivation data from multiple individual reports to create summary plots of *D* vs. temperature. An example for heat inactivation of coronaviruses in liquids and on surfaces has been reported by Guillier et al. [66]. The portion of the dataset within the temperature range 40°C–70°C has been reproduced as **Figure 1** below. As can be appreciated from this figure, there is

Virus[a]	Temperature (°C)	Inactivation matrix	Inactivation efficacy	Reference
SARS-CoV-2	56	Culture medium	3.4 $\log_{10}$ in 15 min	[51]
	65	Culture medium	>6 $\log_{10}$ in 15 min	
SARS-CoV-2	56	Culture medium	4.3 $\log_{10}$ in 10 min	[52]
	70	Culture medium	>5.2 $\log_{10}$ in 10 min	
	90	Culture medium	>5.2 $\log_{10}$ in 10 min	
SARS-CoV-2	56	Culture medium	>3 $\log_{10}$ in 15 min	[53]
	95	Culture medium	>5 $\log_{10}$ in 1 min	
SARS-CoV-2	56	Culture medium	>4 $\log_{10}$ in 30 min	[54]
	65	Culture medium	>4 $\log_{10}$ in 15 min	
SARS-CoV-2	56	Culture medium	>5 $\log_{10}$ in 30 min	[55]
	92	Culture medium	>6 $\log_{10}$ in 2 min	
SARS-CoV-2	56	Culture medium	>5 $\log_{10}$ in 30 min	[56]
	98	Culture medium	>5 $\log_{10}$ in 2 min	
SARS-CoV	60	Phosphate buffered saline	>4 $\log_{10}$ in 15 min	[57]
SARS-CoV	56	Culture medium	>6 $\log_{10}$ in 90 min	[30]
	67	Culture medium	>6 $\log_{10}$ in 60 min	
	75	Culture medium	>6 $\log_{10}$ in 30 min	
SARS-CoV	56	Culture medium	>5 $\log_{10}$ in 30 min	[58]
	60	Culture medium	>5 $\log_{10}$ in 30 min	
SARS-CoV	56	Culture medium	>4 $\log_{10}$ in 10 min	[15]
	65	Culture medium	>4 $\log_{10}$ in 4 min	
SARS-CoV	58	Culture medium	4.9 $\log_{10}$ in 30 min	[59]
	68	Culture medium	≥4.3 $\log_{10}$ in 10 min	
SARS-CoV	56	Culture medium	>6 $\log_{10}$ in 30 min	[29]
MERS-CoV	56	Culture medium	4 $\log_{10}$ in 24 min	[60]
	65	Culture medium	4 $\log_{10}$ in 1 min	
PEDV	50	Culture medium	1.1 $\log_{10}$ in 60 min	[61]
	60	Culture medium	5 $\log_{10}$ in 30 min	
PEDV	48	Culture medium	1.7 $\log_{10}$ in 10 min	[62]
CaCoV	60	Culture medium	>4 $\log_{10}$ in 15 min	[63]
	80	Culture medium	>4 $\log_{10}$ in 1 min	
MHV	60	Culture medium	>4 $\log_{10}$ in 15 min	[63]
	80	Culture medium	>4 $\log_{10}$ in 1 min	
FIPV (Wt)	54	Culture medium	2 $\log_{10}$ in 15 min	[64]

[a]SARS-CoV-2, severe acute respiratory syndrome coronavirus 2; SARS-CoV, severe acute respiratory syndrome coronavirus; MERS-CoV, Middle East respiratory syndrome coronavirus; PEDV, porcine epidemic diarrhea virus; CaCoV, canine coronavirus; MHV, mouse hepatitis virus; FIPV (Wt), feline infectious peritonitis coronavirus (wild-type).

Table 4.
Efficacy of heat inactivation for inactivating coronaviruses in liquid matrices.

Virus[a]	Temperature (°C)	Surface type	Inactivation efficacy	Reference
SARS-CoV-2	70	N95 mask fabric	3 $\log_{10}$ in 48 min	[40]
	70	stainless steel	3 $\log_{10}$ in 88 min	
SARS-CoV-2	70	N95 mask fabric	>5.5 $\log_{10}$ in 60 min	[71]
SARS-CoV-2	55	stainless steel	1 $\log_{10}$ in 35 min	[72]
PEDV	60	N95 mask fabric	≥3 $\log_{10}$ in 20 min	[73]

[a]*SARS-CoV-2, severe acute respiratory syndrome coronavirus 2; PEDV, porcine epidemic diarrhea virus.*

Table 5.
Efficacy of heat inactivation for inactivating coronaviruses on surfaces.

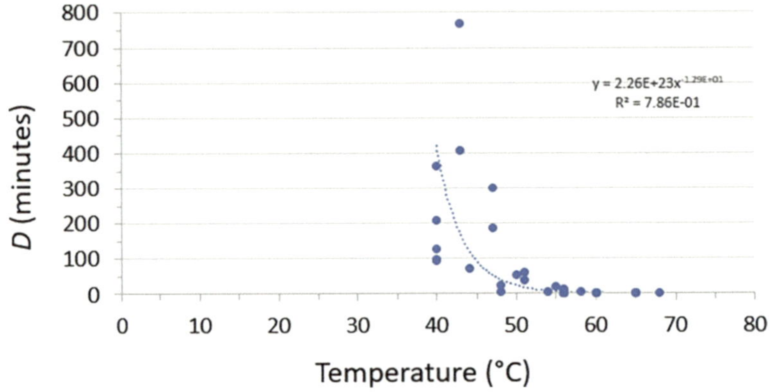

Figure 1.
Relationship between decimal reduction value (D; time required for 1 $\log_{10}$ inactivation) and temperature for heating studies involving various coronaviruses. Data are from reference [66].

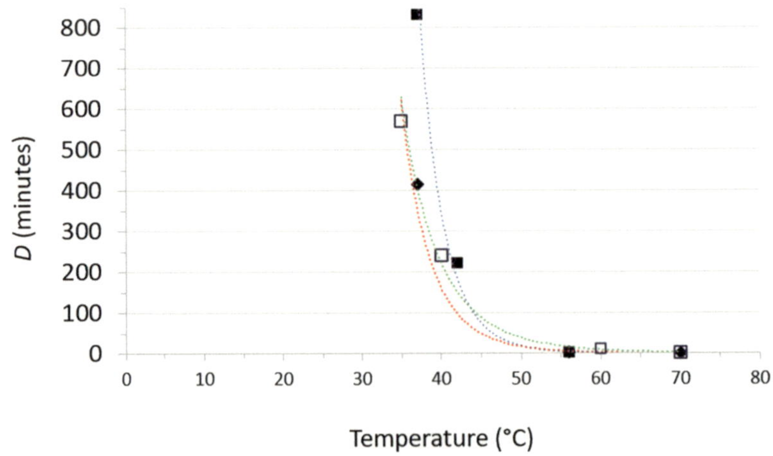

Figure 2.
Relationship between decimal reduction value (D; time required for 1 $\log_{10}$ inactivation) and temperature for heating studies involving SARS-CoV-2. Data are from reference [75] (□), [76] (◆), and [77] ■).

considerable variability in response at the lower temperatures, while greater concurrence is seen at temperatures of 50°C and above. The ability of the power function ($D = a \times \text{temperature}^{-b}$; where D is the decimal reduction value and a and b are calculated coefficients) to fit the combined coronavirus dataset is similar to

Coronavirus	*a*[a]	*b*	r^2	*D* at 56°C (min)	*Reference for D values*
Various *Coronaviridae*	2.26E+23	12.9	0.786	6.4	[66]
Alphacoronaviruses					
TGEV	4.38E+20	10.9	0.967	39	[78]
CaCoV	1.23E+09	4.92	0.856	3.1	[79]
PEDV	7.11E+15	8.57	0.953	7.4	[80]
Betacoronavirus					
SARS-CoV-2	2.70E+18	10.1	0.985	6.0	[76]
SARS-CoV-2	2.97E+23	13.1	0.996	3.7	[77]
SARS-CoV-2	9.52E+6	3.69	0.980	3.4	[51]
SARS-CoV-2 (modeled)	7.18E+14	7.81	0.998	16	[75]

[a]*Abbreviations used:* a *and* b, *coefficients for power function line equation* D = a × *Temperature;* D, *decimal reduction value; CaCoV, canine coronavirus; PEDV, porcine epidemic diarrhea virus; SARS-CoV-2, severe acute respiratory syndrome coronavirus 2; TGEV, transmissible gastroenteritis virus.*

Table 6.
Power function coefficients for D *vs. temperature curves for thermal inactivation of coronaviruses.*

the ability of this function to fit data for multiple temperatures for SARS-CoV-2 generated within a given laboratory (**Figure 2**).

In cases where a laboratory has generated *D* vs. temperature data for three or more temperatures, these data may be plotted as shown in **Figure 2**. This figure compiles line fit data from two empirical liquid inactivation studies for SARS-CoV-2 [76, 77]. The third line on this plot is the line fit obtained from modeling of SARS-CoV-2 inactivation at various temperature by Yap et al. [75]. The modeling by Yap and coworkers was performed on the basis of heat inactivation data generated by various labs, using as challenge viruses a variety of coronaviruses (SARS-CoV, SARS-CoV-2, MERS-CoV, MHV, PEDV, and TGEV) [75]. The agreement between the line fits for these three datasets in striking. It is apparent from the plots in **Figure 2** that it takes hours to achieve 1 $\log_{10}$ inactivation of SARS-CoV-2 at temperatures ≤40°C, while inactivation at temperatures greater than 50°C requires only min.

In **Table 6**, the power function line fit coefficients for heat inactivation studies evaluating various coronaviruses are displayed. The estimation of *D* at 56°C is shown as a means of demonstrating the utility of the power function line fitting approach for enabling comparison of datasets generated at different laboratories. Note that at 56°C, *D* values for the various coronaviruses range from 3 to 39 min, with the 39 min required for TGEV considered to be atypical.

Taken together, the data in **Figures 1** and **2** and **Tables 4–6** support the expectation that similar heat sensitivities are to be expected for various members of the *Coronaviridae* family. To put the *D* values shown in **Table 6** into perspective, more heat susceptible virus families include the *Rhabdoviridae* ($D_{56\ °C}$ ranging from 0.2 to 1.9 min) and *Retroviridae* ($D_{56\ °C}$ of 1.4 min), while less susceptible viruses include animal members of the *Parvoviridae* ($D_{56\ °C}$ > 10 hours) [6]. The heat susceptibilities displayed by the *Coronaviridae* are fairly typical of enveloped and non-enveloped viruses in general, except as noted above.

The literature that has been reviewed above indicate that heat inactivation is typically utilized for inactivation of coronaviruses in solutions, but this physical approach has also been used for decontamination of these viruses on surfaces, such as stainless steel and N95 respirator material. In addition, hot (≥63°C), humid (95%

relative humidity) air exposure for 1 hour has been described for decontaminating enveloped RNA virus (bacteriophage Phi6 used as a surrogate for SARS-CoV-2) dried on surfaces within aircraft [81].

6. Discussion

Physical pathogen inactivation approaches have a number of advantages. First among these is the fact that these approaches display efficacy for a broad range of pathogen types, up to and including bacterial and fungal spores. In the hierarchy of pathogen susceptibility to microbicides (sometimes referred to as the Spaulding scale [82]), only infectious proteins (prions) may remain resistant to these physical approaches as normally applied [83, 84]. Per the established hierarchy with regard to viral inactivation [85–88], non-enveloped viruses display much greater susceptibility to microbicides, while enveloped viruses are considered to be among the most susceptible of all pathogens to microbicides. For physical inactivation approaches, this hierarchy may be somewhat different. As mentioned in the introduction to this chapter, the orthogonal physical approaches may display complementary efficacies for different virus families, and efficacy is not solely determined by envelope status or particle size.

Secondly, to a certain extent, the physical approaches require additions of photons to the inactivation matrix, not molecules—as in the case of chemical inactivation. This means that the physical approaches can be used without the necessity of removing the inactivating agent from the inactivation matrix. For example, gamma irradiation can be applied to finished product in sealed containers, ultraviolet irradiation can be applied through glass or plastic tubing, and heat can be applied to containers of liquids. Each of the methods can be applied to surfaces without the need to subsequently remove an inactivating agent.

The first-order behavior of physical inactivation approaches, discussed previously in this chapter, is also a useful attribute. For instance, gamma irradiation and UVC inactivation efficacies are typically first-order with respect to applied fluence. Efficacy of heat inactivation is typically first-order with respect to time at any given temperature. This means that once a *log_{10} inactivation per fluence* value is obtained, efficacy at a different fluence (gamma irradiation or UVC) can be estimated. Similarly, once a *D* value is obtained at a given temperature for heat inactivation, the efficacy for a different contact time can be estimated with some confidence.

In this chapter, we have attempted to convert, where possible, inactivation results from different reports into the *log_{10} inactivation per fluence* values and the *D* values discussed above, so that the readers can make informed estimates of inactivation efficacy for these approaches under non-evaluated conditions. These estimates are quite straightforward in the case of gamma and UVC irradiation. For example, if 2 log_{10} inactivation per kGy gamma irradiation or per mJ/cm^2 UVC is measured in a study, then 4 log_{10} inactivation should be expected at 2 kGy or at 2 mJ/cm^2. For heat inactivation, if the *D* value at 65°C is 10 min, then 2 log_{10} inactivation should be expected after 20 min at the same temperature. The equations for the power function line fit of *D* vs. temperature plots [6] also allow one to estimate inactivation efficacy for non-measured temperatures. The plots shown in **Figures 1** and **2** can be thought of as depicting a 1 log_{10} inactivation *surface*. Any point on the line reflects the conditions necessary to achieve 1 log_{10} inactivation. Points to the right of this line will result in greater than 1 log_{10} inactivation, while points to the left of the line will result in less than 1 log_{10} inactivation.

As is apparent from this chapter, the three physical inactivation approaches discussed (gamma irradiation, UVC irradiation, and heat inactivation) each display efficacy for all members of the *Coronaviridae* family and for SARS-CoV-2 in particular. The different approaches may be useful, in particular, for different applications. For instance, in case of IPAC, of the three approaches, UVC is most useful for decontaminating indoor air. For such an application, indoor air to be recirculated is passed through a unit which exposes the air to an appropriate UVC fluence. This can be done while the indoor spaces are being occupied. For surface inactivation, each of the three approaches may be useful, depending upon the surface to be decontaminated. For decontamination of liquid matrices, again, each of the three approaches could be useful. The disadvantages of the three approaches are:

- Gamma irradiation. Gamma irradiation must be performed at an irradiation facility. It is typically applied to inanimate surfaces, such as plasticware, at high fluences for sterilization. For decontaminating biological liquids, the irradiation is typically done at low temperature to avoid the damaging effects of indirect radiation effects.

- UVC irradiation. Ultraviolet light is a line-of sight-approach. If the inactivation matrix is shielded from the photons, or absorbs the photons, the efficacy for inactivation will be low. Establishing dosimetry under the actual inactivation conditions and assuring that all portions of the matrix receive photons is essential for efficacy. For IPAC, surface disinfection by UVC must be conducted while the indoor spaces are not occupied.

- Heat inactivation. Extent of inactivation depends on the temperature applied and the contact time, as well as on the specific virus being inactivated. Since coronaviruses appear to be very susceptible to heat inactivation, this approach is useful. Achieving and maintaining the desired inactivation temperature for the required contact time can be challenging. Heat and humidity have been used for IPAC, specifically for disinfecting aircraft cabins [81]. This approach also is commonly applied in the biologics industries.

For each of these physical approaches, a balance must be achieved between the desired $\log_{10}$ reduction in infectious virus level and the need to retain the desired attributes of the material being decontaminated. This includes inanimate surfaces, such as plasticware in the case of gamma irradiation [11]. To put this in another way, users are not always free to use extremely high fluences of gamma or UVC radiation, or extremely high temperatures as a means of assuring decontamination. Each of these physical approaches are capable of causing unintended damage to biological solutions and material surfaces. Treatment of indoor spaces with UVC radiation must be conducted when those spaces are unoccupied by humans.

7. Conclusions

This chapter represents a review of the literature on physical inactivation of SARS-CoV-2 and other members of the *Coronaviridae*. While physical approaches include X-irradiation, electron beam irradiation, and high pressure treatment, literature on those approaches for inactivation of coronaviruses were not identified during the search. Therefore, the chapter discusses only gamma irradiation, UVC irradiation, and heat inactivation. The *Coronaviridae* in general, and SARS-CoV-2 in particular, appear to be quite susceptible to each of these three physical inactivation approaches. The various approaches have utility for different applications. For instance, of the three approaches, UVC is most useful for indoor air decontamination, each is useful for liquid or surface inactivation. Each approach has its advantages and disadvantages, which were discussed for the benefit of the reader.

Acknowledgements

No funding was obtained for conduct of this literature review. The authors thank Dr. M. Khalid Ijaz for constructive review of the manuscript.

Conflict of interest

The authors declare no conflict of interest.

Author details

Raymond W. Nims[1*] and Mark Plavsic[2]

1 RMC Pharmaceutical Solutions, Inc., Longmont, CO, USA

2 Fate Therapeutics, San Diego, CA, USA

*Address all correspondence to: rnims@rmcpharma.com

References

[1] Nims RW, Plavsic M. Efficacy of electron beam for viral inactivation. Journal of Microbial and Biochemical Technology. 2015;7:173-176

[2] Govaris A, Pexara A. Inactivation of foodborne viruses by high-pressure processing (HPP). Foods. 2021;**10**:215. DOI: 10.3390/foods10020215

[3] Anelich LECM, Lues R, Farber JM, Parriera VR. SARS-CoV-2 and risk to food safety. Frontiers in Nutrition. 2020;7:580551. DOI: 10.3389/fnut.2020.580551

[4] Nims RW, Gauvin G, Plavsic M. Gamma irradiation of animal sera for inactivation of viruses and mollicutes: A review. Biologicals. 2011;**39**:370-377

[5] Kowalski WJ, Bahnfleth WP, Hernandez MT. A genomic model for predicting the ultraviolet susceptibility of viruses. IUVA News. 2009;**11**:15-28

[6] Nims RW, Plavsic M. Intra-family and inter-family comparisons for viral susceptibility to heat inactivation. Journal of Microbial and Biochemical Technology. 2013;5:136-141

[7] Nims R, Plavsic M. Identification of worst-case model viruses for selected viral clearance steps. BioProcessing Journal. 2014;**13**:6-13

[8] Brown S, Croonenborghs B, Head K, Senescu M, Nims R, Plavsic M, et al. Gamma irradiation of animal serum: Maintaining the cold chain throughout the process. BioProcessing Journal. 2018;**17**. DOI: 10.12665/J17OA.Brown

[9] Meunier SM, Sasges MR, Aucoin MG. Evaluating ultraviolet sensitivity of adventitious agents in biopharmaceutical manufacturing. Journal of Industrial and Microbiological Biotechnology. 2017;**44**:893-909

[10] Harris RE, Coleman PH, Morahan PS. Stability of minute virus of mice to chemical and physical agents. Applied Microbiology. 1974;**28**:351-354

[11] Hemmerich K, Fitzgerald R, Hallett D, Nims R, Versteegen R. Gamma irradiation of animal serum: theoretical basis of impacts of gamma irradiation on biological and synthetic polymers. BioProcessing Journal. 2019;**18**

[12] Leung A, Tran K, Audet J, Lavineway S, Bastien N, Krishnan J. In vitro inactivation of SARS-CoV-2 using gamma irradiation. ABSA International. 2020;**25**(3):157-160. DOI: 10.1177/1535676020934242

[13] Jain R, Sarkale P, Mali D, Shete AM, Patil DY, Majumdar T, et al. Inactivation of SARS-CoV-2 by gamma irradiation. Indian Journal of Medical Research. 2021. DOI: 10.4103/ijmr.IJMR_2789_20

[14] Feldmann F, Shupert WL, Haddock E, Twardoski B, Feldmann H. Gamma irradiation as an effective method for inactivation of emerging viral pathogens. American Journal of Tropical Medicine and Hygiene. 2019; **100**(5):1275-1277. DOI: 10.4269/ajtmh.18-0937

[15] Darnell MER, Subbarao K, Feinstone SM, Taylor DR. Inactivation of the coronavirus that induces severe acute respiratory syndrome, SARS-CoV. Journal of Virological Methods. 2004; **121**:85-91. DOI: 10.1016/j.jviromet.2004.06.006

[16] Kumar M, Mazur S, Ork BL, Postnikova E, Hensley LE, Jahrling PB, et al. Inactivation and safety testing of Middle East respiratory syndrome coronavirus. Journal of Virological Methods. 2015;**223**:13-18. DOI: 10.1016/j.jviromet.2015.07.002

[17] Abolaban FA, Djouider FM. Gamma irradiation-mediated inactivation of enveloped viruses with conservation of genome integrity: potential application for SARS-CoV-2 inactivated vaccine development. Open Life Sciences. 2021; **16**:558-570

[18] Rathnasinghe R, Jangra S, Miorin L, Schotsaert M, Yahnke C, Garcia-Sastre A. The virucidal effects of 405 nm visible light on SARS-CoV-2 and influenza A virus. Scientific Reports. 2021;**11**:19470. DOI: 10.1038/s41598-021-97797-0

[19] Boegel SJ, Gabriel M, Sasges M, Petri B, D'Agostino MR, et al. Robust evaluation of ultraviolet-C sensitivity for SARS-CoV-2 and surrogate coronaviruses. Microbiology Spectrum. 2021;**9**(2):e00537-e00521. DOI: 10.1128/Spectrum.00537-21

[20] Hadi J, Dunowska M, Wu S, Brightwell G. Control measures for SARS-CoV-2: A review on light-based inactivation of single-stranded RNA viruses. Pathogens. 2020;**9**:737. DOI: 10.3390/pathogens9090737

[21] Pendyala B, Patras A, Pokharel B, D'Souza D. Genomic modeling as an approach to identify surrogates for use in experimental validation of SARS-CoV-2 and HuNoV inactivation by UV-C treatment. Frontiers in Microbiology. 2020;**11**:572331. DOI: 10.3389/fmicb.2020.572331

[22] Patterson EI, Prince T, Anderson ER, Casas-Sanchez A, Smith SL, Cansado-Utrilla C, et al. Methods of inactivation of SARS-CoV-2 for downstream biological assays. Journal of Infectious Diseases. 2020;**222**: 1462-1467

[23] Storm N, McKay LGA, Downs SN, Johnson RI, Birru D, de Samber M, et al. Rapid and complete inactivation of SARS-CoV-2 by ultraviolet-C irradiation. Scientific Reports. 2020;**10**: 22421. DOI: 10.1038/s41598-020-79600-8

[24] Biasin M, Bianco M, Pareschi G, Cavalleri A, Cavatorta C, Fenizia C, et al. UV-C irradiation is highly effective in inactivating SARS-CoV-2 replication. Scientific Reports. 2021;**11**:6260. DOI: 10.1038/s41598-021-85425-w

[25] Inagaki H, Saito A, Sugiyama H, Okabayashi T, Fujimoto S. Rapid inactivation of SARS-CoV-2 with deep-UV LED irradiation. Emerging Microbes & Infections. 2020;**9**. DOI: 10.1080/22221751.2020.1796529

[26] Heilingloh CS, Aufderhorst UW, Schipper L, Dittmer U, Witzke O, Yang D, et al. Susceptibility of SARS-CoV-2 to UV irradiation. American Journal of Infection Control. 2020;**48**:1273-1275

[27] Minamikawa T, Koma T, Suzuki A, Mizuno T, Nagamatsu K, Arimochi H, et al. Quantitative evaluation of SARS-CoV-2 inactivation using a deep ultraviolet light-emitting diode. Scientific Reports. 2021;**11**:5070. DOI: 10.1038/s41598-021-84592-0

[28] Sabino CP, Sellera FP, Sales-Medina DF, Machado RRG, Durigon EL, Freitas-Junior LH, et al. UV-C (254 nm) lethal doses for SARS-CoV-2. Photodiagnosis and Photodynamic Therapy. 2020;**32**: 101995. DOI: 10.1016/j.pdpdt.2020.101995

[29] Kariwa H, Fujii N, Takashima I. Inactivation of SARS coronavirus by means of povidone-iodine, physical conditions and chemical reagents. Dermatology. 2006;**212**(suppl. 1): 119-123

[30] Duan S-M, Zhao X-S, Wen R-F, Huang J-J, Pi G-H, Zhang S-X, et al. Stability of SARS coronavirus in human specimens and environment and its sensitivity to heating and UV irradiation. Biomedical and

Environmental Sciences. 2003;**16**: 246-255

[31] Ma B, Linden YS, Gundy PM, Gerba CP, Sobsey MD, Linden KG. Inactivation of coronaviruses and phage Phi6 from irradiation across UVC wavelengths. Environmental Science & Technology Letters. 2021;**8**(5):425-430

[32] Gerchman Y, Mamane H, Friedman N, Mandelboim M. UV-LED disinfection of coronavirus: wavelength effect. Journal of Photochemistry and Photobiology. B. 2020;**212**:112044. DOI: 10.1016/j.jphotobiol.2020.112044

[33] Rozenberg Y, Lowentahl A. Can we use adenovirus validated ultraviolet systems for inactivation of SARS-CoV-2, the virus that causes COVID-19? Water ONLINE. 2020. Available from: https://www.wateronline.com/doc/can-we-use-adenovirus-validated-uv-systems-cov-the-virus-that-causes-covid-0001

[34] Kitagawa H, Nomura T, Nazmul T, Omori K, Shigemoto N, Sakaguchi T, et al. Effect5iveness of 222-nm ultraviolet light on disinfecting SARS-CoV-2 surface contamination. American Journal of Infection Control. 2021;**49**: 299-301

[35] Fischer RJ, Morris DH, van Doremalen N, Sarchette S, Matson MJ, Bushmaker T, et al. Effectiveness of N95 respirator decontamination and reuse against SARS-CoV-2 virus. Emerging Infectious Diseases. 2020;**26**(9): 2253-2255

[36] Buonanno M, Welch D, Shuryak I, Brenner DJ. Far-UVC light (222 nm) efficiently and safely inactivates airborne human coronaviruses. Scientific Reports. 2020;**10**:10285. DOI: 10.1038/s41598-020-67211-2

[37] Walker CM, Ko G. Effect of ultraviolet germicidal irradiation on viral aerosols. Environmental Science and Technology. 2007;**41**:5460-5465

[38] Deshmukh DR, Pomeroy BD. Ultraviolet inactivation and photoreactivation of avian viruses. Avian Diseases. 1969;**13**(**3**):596-602

[39] Chiappa F, Frascella B, Vigezzi GP, Moro M, Diamanti L, Gentile L, et al. The efficacy of ultraviolet light-emitting technology against coronaviruses: A systematic review. Journal of Hospital Infection. 2021;**114**:63-78

[40] Helßling M, Hönes K, Vatter P, Lingenfelder C. Ultraviolet irradiation doses for coronavirus inactivation: Review and analysis of coronavirus photoinactivation studies. GMS Hygiene and Infection Control. 2020;**15**

[41] Bedell K, Buchaklian A, Perlman S. Efficacy of an automated multi-emitter whole room UV-C disinfection system against coronaviruses MHV and MERS-CoV. Infection Control and Hospital Epidemiology. 2016;**37**(5):598-599

[42] Hitchman M. A new perspective of the chemistry and kinetics of inactivation of COVID-19 coronavirus aerosols. Future Virology. 2021;**15**(12): 823-835

[43] Buchan AG, Yang L, Atkinson KD. Predicting airborne coronavirus inactivation by far-UVC in populated rooms using a high-fidelity coupled radiation-CFD model. Scientific Reports. 2020;**10**:19659. DOI: 10.1038/s41598-020-76597-y

[44] de Abajo FJG, Hernández RJ, Kaminer I, Meyerhans A, Rosell-Llompart J, Sanchez-Elsner T. Back to normal: An old physics route to reduce SARS-CoV-2 transmission in indoor spaces. ACS Nano. 2020;**14**(7): 7704-7713

[45] Criscuolo E, Diotti RA, Ferrarese R, Alippi C, Viscardi G, Signorelli C, et al. Fast inactivation of SARS-CoV-2 by UV-C and ozone exposure on different materials. Emerging Microbes &

Infections. 2021;**10**. DOI: 10.1080/22221751.2021.1872354

[46] Rathnasinghe R, Karlicek RF Jr, Schotsaert M, Koffas M, Arduini BL, Jangra S, et al. Scalable, effective, and rapid decontamination of SARS-CoV-2 contaminated N95 respirators using germicidal ultraviolet C (UVC) irradiation device. Scientific Reports. 2021;**1**:19970. DOI: 10.1038/s41598-021-99431-5

[47] Derraik JGB, Anderson WA, Connelly EA, Anderson YC. Rapid review of SARS-CoV-1 and SARS-CoV-2 viability, susceptibility to treatment, and the disinfection and reuse of PPE, particularly filtering facepiece respirators. International Journal of Environmental Research and Public Health. 2020;**17**(17):6117. DOI: 10.3390/ijerph17176117

[48] Zhou SS, Wilde C, Chen Z, Kapes T, Purgill J, Nims R, et al. Carrier and liquid heat inactivation of poliovirus and adenovirus. In: Disinfection. London, UK: InTech; 2018. p. 76340

[49] Zhou SS, Wilde C, Chen Z, Kapes T, Purgill J, Nims, et al. Thermal inactivation of feline calicivirus and herpes simplex virus type 1: side-by-side suspension and carrier studies. Integrative Journal of Veterinary Biosciences 2020;**4**:1-6.

[50] Nims R, Zhou SS, Plavsic M. Identification of worst-case model viruses for low and high pH inactivation. BioProcessing Journal. 2017;**16**:7-14

[51] Batéjat C, Grassin Q, Manuguerra J-C, Leclercq I. Heat inactivation of the severe acute respiratory syndrome coronavirus 2. Journal of Biosafety and Biosecurity. 2021;**3**:1-3. DOI: 10.1016/j.jobb.2020.12.001

[52] Xiling G, Yin C, Ling W, Xiaosong W, Jingjing F, Fang L, et al. In vitro inactivation of SARS-CoV-2 by commonly used disinfection products and methods. Scientific Reports. 2021;**11**:2418

[53] Burton J, Love H, Richards K, Burton C, Summers S, Pitman J, et al. The effect of heat-treatment on SARS-CoV-2 viability and detection. Journal of Virological Methods. 2021;**290**:114087. DOI: 10.1016/j.jviromet.2021.114087

[54] Kim Y-I, Casel MAB, Kim S-M, Kim S-G, Park S-J, Kim E-H, et al. Development of severe acute respiratory syndrome coronavirus 2 (SARS-CoV-2) thermal inactivation method with preservation of diagnostic sensitivity. Journal of Microbiology. 2020;**58**(10):886-891

[55] Pastorino B, Touret F, Gilles M, de Lamballerie X, Charrel RN. Heat inactivation of different types of SARS-CoV-2 samples: What protocols for biosafety, molecular detection and serological diagnostics? Viruses. 2020;**12**:735

[56] Auerswald H, Yann S, Dul S, In S, Dussart P, Martin NJ, et al. Assessment of inactivation procedures for SARS-CoV-2. Journal of General Virology. 2021;**102**:001539. DOI: 10.1099/jgv.0.001539

[57] Darnell MER, Taylor DR. Evaluation of inactivation methods for severe acute respiratory syndrome coronavirus in noncellular blood products. Transfusion. 2006;**46**:1770-1777

[58] Rabenau HF, Cinatl J, Morgenstern B, Bauer G, Preiser W, Doerr HW. Stability and inactivation of SARS coronavirus. Medical and Microbiological Immunology. 2005;**194**:1-6

[59] Pagat A-M, Seux-Goepfert R, Lutsch C, Lecouturier V, Saluzzo J-F, Kusters IC. Evaluation of SARS-coronavirus decontamination procedures. Applied Biosafety. 2007;**12**(2):100-108

[60] Leclercq I, Batéjat C, Burguière AM, Manuguerra J-C. Heat inactivation of the Middle East respiratory syndrome coronavirus. Influenza and Other Respiratory Viruses. 2014;**8**(5):585-586

[61] Hofmann M, Wyler R. Quantitation, biological and physicochemical properties of cell culture-adapted porcine epidemic diarrhea coronavirus (PEDV). Veterinary Microbiology. 1989;**20**:131-142

[62] Hulst MM, Heres L, Hakze-van der Honing RW, Pelser M, Fox M. van der Poel WHM. Study on inactivation of porcine epidemic diarrhea virus, porcine sapelovirus 1 and adenovirus in the production and storage of laboratory spray-dried porcine plasma. Journal of Applied Microbiology. 2019;**126**: 1931-1943

[63] Saknimit M, Inatsuki I, Sugiyama Y, Yagami K-i. Virucidal efficacy of physico-chemical treatments against coronaviruses and parvoviruses of laboratory animals. Jikken Dobutsu. 1988;**37**(3):341-345

[64] Christianson KK, Ingersoll JD, Landon RM, Pfieffer NE, Gerber JD. Characterization of a temperature sensitive feline infectious peritonitis coronavirus. Archives of Virology. 1989; **109**:185-196

[65] Millar BC, Moore JE. Re-purposing of domestic steam disinfectors within the Hospital-at-Home setting: reconciliation of steam disinfector thermal performance against SARS-CoV-2 (COVID-19), norovirus and other viruses' thermal susceptibilities. Infection, Disease & Health. 2021;**26**: 156-159

[66] Guillier L, Martin-Latil S, Chaix E, Thébault A, Pavio N, Le Poder S, et al. Modeling the inactivation of viruses from the Coronaviridae family in response to temperature and relative humidity in suspensions or on surfaces. Applied and Environmental Microbiology. 2020;**86**(18):e01244-e01220. DOI: 10.1128/AEM.01244-20

[67] Kampf G, Voss A, Scheithauer S. Inactivation of coronaviruses by heat. Journal of Hospital Infection. 2020;**105**: 348-349

[68] Jiang Y, Zhang H, Wippold JA, Gupta J, Dai J, de Figueiredo P, et al. Sub-second heat inactivation of coronavirus using a betacoronavirus model. Biotechnology and Bioengineering. 2021;**118**(5):2067-2075

[69] Biryukov J, Boydston JA, Dunning RA, Yeager JJ, Wood S, Reese AL, et al. Increasing temperature and relative humidity accelerates inactivation of SARS-CoV-2 on surfaces. mSphere. 2020;**5**(4):e00441-e00420. DOI: 10.1128/mSphere.00441-20

[70] Morris DH, Yinda KC, Gamble A, Rossine FW, Huang Q, Bushmaker T, et al. Mechanistic theory predicts the effects of temperature and humidity on inactivation of SARS-CoV-2 and other enveloped viruses. eLife. 2021;**10**: e65902

[71] Singh G, Jorgenson J, Pringle T, Nelson T, Ramamoorthy S. Monitoring SARS-CoV-2 decontamination by dry heat and ultraviolet treatment with a swine coronavirus as a surrogate. Infection Prevention in Practice. 2021;**3**:100103. DOI: 10.1016/j.infpip. 2020.100103

[72] Biryukov J, Boydston JA, Dunning RA, Yeager JJ, Wood S, Ferris A, et al. SARS-CoV-2 is rapidly inactivated at high temperature. Environmental Chemistry Letters. 2021;**19**:1773-1777

[73] Daeschler SC, Manson N, Joachim K, Chin AWH, Chan K, Chen PZ, et al. Effect of moist heat reprocessing of N95 respirators on SARS-CoV-2 inactivation and respirator function. CMAJ. 2020; **192**:E1189-E1197

[74] Nims R, Plavsic M. A proposed modeling approach for comparing the heat inactivation susceptibility of viruses. Bioprocessing Journal. 2013; **12**(2):25-35

[75] Yap TF, Liu Z, Shveda RA, Preston DJ. A predictive model of the temperature-dependent inactivation of coronaviruses. Applied Physics Letters. 2020;**117**:060601. DOI: doi.org/10.1063/5.0020782

[76] Chin AWH, Chu JTS, Perera MRA, Hui KPY, Yen H-L, Chan MCW, et al. Stability of SARS-CoV-2 in different environmental conditions. The Lancet Microbe. 2020;**1**(1):e10. DOI: 10.1016/S2666-5247(20)30003-3

[77] Wang TT, Lien CZ, Liu S, Selvaraj P. Effective heat inactivation of SARS-CoV-2. medRxiv (preprint). 2020. DOI: 10.1101/2020.04.29.20085498

[78] Laude H. Thermal inactivation studies of a coronavirus, transmissible gastroenteritis virus. Journal of General Virology. 1981;**56**:235-240

[79] Pratelli A. Canine coronavirus inactivation with physical and chemical agents. The Veterinary Journal. 2008; **177**:71-79

[80] Quist-Rybachuk GV, Nauwynck HJ, Kalmar ID. Sensitivity of porcine epidemic diarrhea virus (PEDV) to pH and heat treatment in the presence or absence of porcine plasma. Veterinary Microbiology. 2015; **181**(3–4):283-288

[81] Buhr TL, Young AA, Borgers-Klonkowski E, Kennihan NL, Barnette HK, Minter ZA, et al. Hot, humid air decontamination of aircraft confirmed that high temperature and high humidity are critical for inactivation of infectious enveloped ribonucleic acid (RNA) virus. Frontiers in Bioengineering and Biotechnology. 2020;**8**:592621. DOI: 10.3389/fbioe.2020.592621

[82] United States Environmental Protection Agency. Office of Pesticide Programs. Final Summary of the Disinfection Hierarchy Workshop. 2016. Available from: https://www.epa.gov/sites/production/files/2016-02/documents/dh_final_summary_of_workshop_-exploration_of_the_disinfection_hierarchy_meeting_summary_final_docx_2_4_16.pdf

[83] Taylor DM. Inactivation of prions by physical and chemical means. Journal of Hospital Infection. 1999;**43**(suppl 1): S69-S76

[84] Giles K, Woerman AL, Berry DB, Prusiner SB. Bioassays and inactivation of prions. Cold Spring Harbor Perspectives in Biology. 2017;**9**(8): a023499. DOI: 10.1101/cshperspect.a023499

[85] Klein M, Deforest A. Principles of viral inactivation. In: Block SS, editor. Disinfection, Sterilization, and Peservation. 3rd ed. Philadelphia: Lea and Febiger; 1983. pp. 422-434

[86] Sattar SA. Hierarchy of susceptibility of viruses to environmental surface disinfectants: A predictor of activity against new and emerging viral pathogens. Journal of the AOAC International. 2007;**90**(6): 1655-1658

[87] Ijaz MK, Rubino JR. Should test methods for disinfectants use vertebrate virus dried on carriers to advance virucidal claims? Infection Control and Hospital Epidemiology. 2008;**29**(2): 192-194

[88] Ijaz MK, Sattar SA, Rubino JR, Nims RW, Gerba CP. Combating SARS-CoV-2: leveraging microbicidal experiences with other emerging/re-emerging viruses. PeerJ. 2020;**8**:e9914. DOI: 10.7717/peerj.9914

Section 3

Viral Persistence and Disinfection

Chapter 8

Environmental Persistence of SARS-CoV-2 and Disinfection of Work Surfaces in View of Pandemic Outbreak of COVID-19

Koushlesh Ranjan

Abstract

Coronavirus disease 2019 (COVID-19) is primarily a respiratory illness, caused by severe acute respiratory syndrome coronavirus 2 (SARS-CoV-2). The pandemic outbreak of SARS-CoV-2 across the world has been responsible for high morbidity and mortality, which emphasizes the role of the environment on virus persistence and propagation to the human population. Since environmental factors may play important roles in viral outbreaks, and the severity of the resulting diseases, it is essential to take into account the role of the environment in the COVID-19 pandemic. The SARS-CoV-2 may survive outside the human body from a few hours to a few days, depending upon environmental conditions, probably due to the relatively fragile envelope of the virus. The shedding and persistence of SARS-CoV-2 in the environment on animate and inanimate objects contributes to the risk of indirect transmission of the virus to healthy individuals, emphasizing the importance of various disinfectants in reducing the viral load on environmental surface and subsequently control of SARS-CoV-2 in the human population.

Keywords: SARS-CoV-2, disinfection, inactivation, surfaces, nanotechnology

1. Introduction

The causative agent of coronavirus disease-19 (COVID-19), the Betacoronavirus, severe acute respiratory syndrome coronavirus 2 (SARS-CoV-2), was for the first time isolated in Wuhan, China in December 2019, from a patient suffering from non-recognizable acute pneumonia [1]. Subsequently, COVID-19 and the causative virus have spread to different regions of the globe, with the greatest number of caseloads being observed in the industrialized countries. Betacoronaviruses belong to the family Coronaviridae, which are enveloped viruses with single-stranded RNA genomes with positive polarity. These viruses are responsible for a wide range of infections in humans, primarily of the upper respiratory tract, including pneumonia, bronchitis, bronchiolitis, etc. [2]. The primary route of transmission of SARS-CoV-2 is thought to be contact with oral-nasal droplets released from infected persons during coughing, sneezing, and talking [3]. The transmission of SARS-CoV-2 through food and water has not yet been well established. Studies on previous epidemics caused by Middle East respiratory syndrome coronavirus (MERS-CoV) and severe acute respiratory syndrome coronavirus (SARS-CoV) have identified no cases of viral transmission through food. Similarly, no cases of transmission of SARS-CoV-2 infections via food have been identified [4]. Therefore, SARS-CoV-2 is not recognized as a foodborne virus and the risk of transmission of COVID-19 through contaminated food is considered to be very low [4]. On the other hand, studies have demonstrated the presence of viral genetic material in the blood and anal swabs from human patients [5]. The fact that diarrhea is a symptom of COVID-19 raises concerns about possible transmission of SARS-CoV-2 via the fecal-oral route. Destite this, it is not yet clear that the fecal-oral route represents a significant transmission modality for this virus [6].

Fortunately, the lipid envelope of this virus renders it susceptible to a wide variety of disinfectants. As such, this virus is expected to be more susceptible to inactivation by microbicides in comparison to non-enveloped viruses with a similar route of transmission, such as norovirus, adenovirus, hepatitis A virus, etc. [7, 8]. Several physical agents, such as sunlight, high temperature, UV radiation, and gamma radiation, etc. also act as effective agents to inactivate the virus [9]. SARS-CoV-2 exhibits temperature sensitivity and can be inactivated within 5 minutes at 70°C [9]. Healthcare areas contain several types of high-touch environmental surfaces, including furniture, tables, chairs, and toilets, along with medical instruments, including stethoscopes, wheelchairs, incubators, etc. [10]. These environmental surfaces are vulnerable to contamination with SARS-CoV-2 shed from patients [11, 12].

Previous studies have confirmed that SARS-CoV-2 transmission is linked with close contact of infected and healthy individuals within a closed setting, such as exists in healthcare facilities and residential institutions, etc. [11]. The same considerations apply to settings outside of the healthcare arena, including temples, churches, mosques, local markets, and business centers, etc. [13].

Transmission of SARS-CoV-2 from infected to healthy individuals may be disrupted through disinfection of contaminated high-touch environmental surfaces. The survivability (persistence of infectivity) of SARS-CoV-2 informs the need for surface disinfection at an appropriate frequency. However, in areas where resources for regular disinfection and cleaning are limited, the guideline should be mandated for avoiding frequent touching of the face along with frequent hand washing to reduce the risk of SARS-CoV-2 transmission associated with surface contamination and transfer of virus from hands to susceptible mucous membranes of the eye, nose, and mouth.

2. SARS-CoV-2 persistence in the environment and risk of transmission to humans

The study of the persistence of SARS-CoV-2 in the environment is necessary, as this informs the need for and frequency of disinfection of those surfaces. This virus shows environmental persistence for a few hours to a few days. Several studies are now available to provide viral persistence data for various environmental surfaces, both porous and non-porous. Many of these studies also documented the virus persistence half-life or decay rate information on different surfaces and materials [9, 14–22]. This information allows one to estimate the amount of time necessary for the virus to decay to titers beneath an estimated human minimal infectious dose. As might be expected, the amount of time required depends, in part, on the initial contamination titer for the surface, the type of surface, and the temperature and relative humidity.

2.1 Environmental and surface persistence of SARS-CoV-2

Previous research work related to the environmental persistence of coronavirus species was conducted on human coronavirus strain HCoV-229E [23]. This virus was found to survive for 2 hours to 9 days on various surfaces including metal, glass, and plastic. Moreover, the study also confirmed the temperature sensitivity of coronaviruses. Environmental temperatures in the range of 30–40°C were found to reduce the persistence of transmissible gastroenteritis virus (TGEV), Middle East respiratory syndrome coronavirus (MERS-CoV), and mouse hepatitis virus (MHV) [23]. At environmental temperatures above 40°C the virus is inactivated within hours to minutes [24]. However, based on the lack of experimental data available on the minimal human infectious doses of the human coronaviruses, it is difficult to say for how long the viruses may survive on different inanimate surfaces at levels actually capable of infecting a human host.

Subsequently, several studies have been conducted on environmental persistence of SARS-CoV-2 specifically (**Table 1**). The data on the survival of SARS-CoV-2 on different surfaces have revealed that viral persistence on prototypic high-touch environmental surfaces (HITES) mainly depends upon four factors: the type of surface (porosity), presence of organic matrix on the surface, temperature/humidity, and time [9, 15–22, 25, 27]. The survival data analyses for SARS-CoV-2 demonstrate that the virus remains infectious for longer durations on hard non-porous surfaces, such as stainless steel and plastic, in comparison with cardboard or wood [15]. The presence of organic matrix during drying of SARS-CoV-2 on surfaces may lead to an increase in half-life of the virus [16, 17, 21]. However, in one of the studies it was demonstrated that SARS-CoV-2 exhibited a shorter half-life on a surface in the presence of human mucus and sputum in comparison to when dried in presence of matrix of culture medium [18]. In the absence of an organic load, the half-life of SARS-CoV-2 on plastic, glass, and aluminum surfaces was demonstrated as 35 hours, 7 hours, and 0.33 hours, respectively at 19–21°C and 45–55% relative humidity (RH) [17]. Similarly, the persistence half-life on stainless steel, wood, in a matrix of 10% suspension of human feces or human urine was demonstrated as 23 hours, 21 hours, 2.6 hours, and 16 hours, respectively at 25–27°C and 35% relative humidity [20]. In another study the persistence of SARS-CoV-2 in human sputum and mucus was found to be very close to that on porous surfaces, with half-lives of 1.9 and 3.5 hours, respectively [18]. These half-life values demonstrate that the SARS-CoV-2 may remain infectious for few days on HITES following a contamination event, if hygiene interventions are not implemented.

In one of the studies, infectious SARS-CoV-2 was detected at up to 10 days on mink fur, 5 days on plastic, 1 day on faux fur, and less than a day on various materials including faux leather, cotton, and polyester [22]. Further study revealed that UV light failed to inactivate the virus on pelts, probably due to mechanical protection by the fur. However, heat treatment at 60°C for 1 h was found sufficient to inactivate the virus on all the mentioned surfaces [22].

Other researchers have also evaluated the environmental persistence of the SARS-CoV-2 on different surfaces. In one such study, it was demonstrated that SARS-CoV-2 remained infectious for up to 1 day on wood and cloth, 2 days on a glass surface, 4 days on stainless steel and plastic surfaces, and up to 7 days on facemasks [9]. Similarly, in another study, it was found that SARS-CoV-2 remained infectious for up to 4 hours on a copper metal surface, 24 hours on a cardboard surface, and 72 hours on objects made of plastic and stainless-steel materials [25].

SARS-CoV-2 infectivity has been found to persist over a wide range of ambient temperatures and pH values, but the virus was found to be susceptible to temperatures above 40°C [24] and standard disinfection procedures (**Table 1**) [15]. The environmental survivability of the virus depends on various factors, such as types of material, surfaces, temperature, and humidity. For instance, it has been shown that SARS-CoV-2 may remain viable for up to 4 hours on a copper surface, and up to 72 hours on a stainless steel or plastic surface (**Table 1**) [25]. Similarly, this virus

S. n.	Surface material	Relative Humidity (%)	Temperature (°C)	Persistence (Minute/ Hour/Day)	Complete inactivation (Hour/Day)	Reference
Porous surfaces						
1	Surgical mask (inner layer)	65	22	4 days	7 days	[9]
2	Surgical mask (outer layer)	65	22	7 d	—	[9]
3	Tissue paper	65	22	30 minutes	3 hours	[9]
4	Cloth	65	22	1 day	2 days	[9]
5	Cotton	35–40	20	1 hour	4 hours	[16]
6	Nitrile Gloves	35–40	20	7 days	7 days	[16]
7	Chemical gloves	35–40	20	4 day	4 days	[16]
8	N95 mask	35–40	20	14 days	21 days	[16]
9	N100 mask	35–40	20	14 days	21 days	[16]
10	Tyvek	35–40	20	14 days	21 days	[16]
11	Wood	65	22	1 day	2 days	[5]
12	Paper	65	22	30 minutes	3 hours	[9]
Non-porous surfaces						
13	Cardboard	65	21–23	1 day	2 days	[25]
14	Copper	65	21–23	4 hours	8 hours	[25]
15	Polypropylene Plastic	65	21–23	3 days	4 days	[25]
16	Banknote paper	65	22	2 days	4 days	[9]
17	Plastics (face shield)	35–40	20	21 days	21 days	[16]
18	Stainless steel	35–40	20	14 days	21 days	[16]
19	Stainless steel	65	21–23	3 days	4 days	[25]
20	Stainless steel	65	22	4 days	7 days	[9]
Liquid medium and Air sample						
21	Aerosol	65	21–23	3 hours	—	[25]
22	Aerosol	53	23	>16 hour	—	[26]
23	Virus transport medium	—	4	14 days	—	[9]
24	Virus transport medium	—	22	—	14 days	[9]
25	Virus transport medium	—	37	—	2 days	[9]
26	Virus transport medium	—	70	—	5 minutes	[9]

Table 1.
Persistence of SARS-CoV-2 on different prototypic environmental surfaces.

may survive for up to 1 day on cloth and wood, 2 days on a glass surface, and up to 7 days on the outer surface of a regular medical mask along with a wide range of ambient temperature and pH values of 3–10 [9]. However, in another study it was demonstrated that the stability of SARS-CoV (a related betacoronavirus) may rapidly decrease after exposure to low pH (pH < 3) and high temperature (>65°C) [28].

The surface viability of SARS-CoV-2 was demonstrated in one of the experiments using plaque assay followed by viral RNA extraction and detection [14]. The study showed that infectious viruses may persist for the longest duration on a surgical mask and stainless steel, with an overall reduction in infectivity of 99.9% by 122 and 114 hours, respectively. On polyester shirt and banknote, the infectivity of SARS-CoV-2 reduced to 99.9% within 2.5 hours and 75 hours, respectively. Further study revealed that SARS-CoV-2 is most stable on nonporous hydrophobic surfaces. The viral RNA was also found highly stable on surfaces, and only 1 $\log_{10}$ reduction in recovery was observed in three weeks [14]. However, in comparison to viral RNA, the infectivity of SARS-CoV-2 reduced more rapidly on surfaces. The level of infectivity SARS-CoV-2 may become undetectable within 2 days on environmental surfaces. This indicates that mere detection of viral RNA on surfaces does not prove the presence of infectious SARS-CoV-2 [14].

Studies have also been conducted to evaluate the survival time of coronaviruses in food matrices. It has been demonstrated that MERS-CoV may survive up to 72 hours in food at 40°C [29]. In a similar study, a lower persistence of human coronavirus 229E (HCoV-229E) was found in comparison to poliovirus 1 (PV-1) on lettuce stored at 40°C [27]. Further, the study revealed that HCoV-229E was not detected on lettuce samples after four days of storage at 40°C and no virus was identified after ten days of spiking of HCoV-229E on another fruit sample (strawberries) [27]. Recent evidence suggests that coronaviruses may remain stable at low temperatures on food and surfaces for an extended period. This suggest that, theoretically, SARS-CoV-2 transmission through foods or food packaging when stored under these conditions [30]. An experimental study under laboratory conditions revealed that SARS-CoV-2 remained highly stable at freezing (−10 to −80°C) and refrigerated (4°C) temperatures on poultry, meat, fish, and swine skin for 14–21 days [30]. Similarly, in another study SARS-CoV-2 was found stable on swine skin even after 14 days at 4°C [19]. These studies suggest that SARS-CoV-2 might remain infectious for a prolonged period in food stored at low temperature. In another study, SARS-CoV-2 was isolated from the swab samples of imported frozen cod outer package surfaces, which showed that the frozen food industry may transmit SARS-CoV-2 virus to other countries and regions [31]. Therefore, based upon available data, it can be hypothesized that contaminated cold-storage foods may pose a risk for SARS-CoV-2 transmission. Since coronaviruses are thermolabile and thus susceptible to traditional heat treatments of cooking (70°C), consumption of cooked foods should not pose risk of transmission of these viruses. Consumption of uncooked or frozen food should be avoided during a coronvirus outbreak to avoid possible transmission of virus.

2.2 SARS-CoV-2 survival on atmospheric particulate matter

Airborne particulate matter may also transmit the causative agent of COVID-19. In hospital wards, SARS-CoV-2 RNA has been recovered from air samples collected in greater amounts than recovered from outdoor premises [32]. The study suggests that air might be a route of virus transmission. The aerosol-generating mechanisms in healthcare facilities are a major cause of concern. For instance, researchers have demonstrated the possibility of airborne diffusion of the virus from aerosols and suspended particles in the air at hospitals in Wuhan (China) [33] and Omaha (USA) [34]. The initial study confirmed the persistence of 1 to 113 genomic copies/m^3 of SARS-CoV-2 in the air in Wuhan Hospital during gatherings of high numbers of people. With the reduction in the number of patients and adequate sanitization and disinfection, viral RNA was not detected [33]. Similarly, at Nebraska Medical Center, Omaha (USA), 63.2% positivity for the presence of SARS-CoV-2 RNA was detected in analyzed air samples, with 2 to 9 genomic copies/L of virus [34].

The atmospheric pollutants and particulate matter (PM_{10} and $PM_{2.5}$) may also be linked with the spread of respiratory viral infections, because particulate matter may act as a carrier (vehicle) for viruses [35]. Researchers have confirmed the increased transmission of SARS-CoV-2 through PM_{10} in Italy [36]. Therefore, it is assumed that air pollution and particulate matter in the air may contribute to the spread of COVID-19. Periodic air monitoring may be needed to mitigate the risk of transmission of the virus in the most highly impacted environments.

2.3 Survival of coronavirus in water and wastewater effluents

The onset of respiratory infections on a large scale in the human population informs the need for detailed information concerning the survival of coronavirus in water and wastewater effluents. The persistence of several coronaviruses, such as feline infectious peritonitis virus (FIPV) and human coronavirus 229E (HCoV-229E), has been analyzed in tap water and wastewater samples [37]. Filtered tap water showed a lesser number of viruses [37]. Moreover, the study also revealed that coronavirus persistence in wastewater depended on temperature and levels of organic matter. To inactivate the coronaviruses in tap water at the level of 99.9% at 23°C, 10 days were required. Further study revealed that these viruses may survive up to 588 days in tap water at 4°C [37]. However, the time required to inactivate the coronaviruses in wastewater plant effluents up to 99.9% varied between 2.3 to 3.5 days at 23°C [37]. This study also revealed that the transmission risk of coronavirus through water is less in comparison to enteroviruses, such as poliovirus 1, due to the faster inactivation of coronaviruses in wastewater effluents at ambient temperature.

However, with the current inactivation and persistence estimates on surrogate viruses, it is difficult to predict the fate of SARS-CoV-2 in water and wastewater. Several researchers have initiated study of SARS-CoV-2 persistence in water and wastewater. In one of the studies, 90% reduction (T_{90}) in infectious SARS-CoV-2 in tap water and wastewater at room temperature was observed after 1.5 and 1.7 days, respectively [38]. However, in wastewater the T_{90} values for infectious SARS-CoV-2 were reported as 15 min and 2 min at 50°C and 70°C, respectively [38]. Researchers have identified SARS-CoV-2 RNA in river water. However, no infectivity detected in cultured cells was observed for the recovered SARS-CoV-2 [39]. As mentioned before, this emphasizes that the identification of viral RNA in the environment does not equate to presence of infectious virus. In another study, it was revealed that SARS-CoV-2 may survive up to 14 days under laboratory conditions at 4°C in a virus transport medium. SARS-CoV-2 was incubated in a virus transport medium at a final concentration ~ 6·8 $\log_{10}$ $TCID_{50}$ per mL at 4°C. After 14 days, there was only a 0·7 $\log_{10}$ reduction in infectious titer observed [9].

2.4 SARS-CoV-2 persistence in hospital and industrial wastewater

Apart from enteric viruses, certain species of coronaviruses may also remain present in wastewater [40]. However, the persistence of SARS-CoV-2 in wastewater and the potential for transmission through the fecal-oral route has yet to be confirmed. The studies have confirmed the inhibiting effect of wastewater on the persistence of coronaviruses [41]. In contrast to this, in one of the studies it was also demonstrated that coronavirus surrogates may survive for a longer duration in non-filtered primary effluents in comparison to filtered samples [37]. The longer survival duration in non-filtered water is primarily attributed to the presence of organic sediments which may provide protection from chemical or biological inactivating agents present in water. In contrast, the available data on surrogate viruses for SARS-COV-2 suggest that the novel coronavirus may be less persistent in wastewater, primarily due to the presence of organic substances as well as inhibiting matrix autochthonous flora, including protozoa, which may contribute proteases and nucleases resulting in faster inactivation of the virus [42].

As a response to the SARS-CoV-2 pandemic and relatively high transmissibility of SARS-CoV-2, several countries have implemented the monitoring of wastewater streams to confirm the presence of the virus in the community, with special reference to asymptomatic individuals and the possibility of risk to contamination of wastewater and risk to solid waste treatment plant employees [43].

SARS-CoV-2 RNA has been detected in human feces [44] and in raw sewage and sludge [45, 46]. The levels correlate with the COVID-19 epidemiological curve and increased number of hospital admissions [46]. Again, the detection of viral RNA does not necessarily indicate the presence of infectious virus particles; rather it indicates the viral prevalence in community.

SARS-CoV-2 RNA was also detected in the wastewater at the Amsterdam Schiphol Airport (Netherlands) and the wastewater treatment plant in Kaatsheuvel (Netherlands) in 2020. This was a crucial finding, since the first case of COVID-19 was reported in February 2020 and viral genetic materials in wastewater samples were detected in March 2020 in Netherland [47]. In one of the studies, SARS-CoV was found to remain infectious at 20°C in wastewater for up to 2 days and viral genomic RNA was isolated for about 8 days [48]. It is not unexpected that SARS-CoV RNA can be detected in wastewater following disinfection protocols using chlorine [48].

Most of these reports are discussing the detection of viral RNA in hospital and sewage water, which does not necessarily confirm the presence of infectious virus. The real challenge is to identify and prevent the transmission of infectious SARS-CoV-2 particles in bioaerosols created during flushing of toilets. Several studies have reported the presence of high concentrations of SARS-CoV-2 in aerosols from patients' toilets and the neighboring environment in hospitals [11, 49, 50]. Thus, toilets may represent one of the most highly contaminated areas of the hospital and may play a potential role in COVID-19 transmission in hospitals. The above studies justify the requirement for adequate disinfection protocols in hospital premises when treating COVID-19 patients, with the aim of inactivating the virus and mitigating possible subsequent spread in hospital wastewater.

2.5 Viral persistence in sewage and biological solids

The possibility of transmission of SARS-CoV-2 from asymptomatic patients via the fecal-oral route is under study. Wastewater-based viral epidemiology and surveillance of sewage material may provide valuable information regarding the prevalence of SARS-CoV-2 in the human population, which may be used as an early warning system in disease forecasting. In biological waste materials and specimens, such as in human serum, plasma, feces, and sputum, SARS-CoV may survive up to 96 hours. However, in human urine, the virus survives for a lesser time, probably due to the presence of urea and adverse pH conditions [51]. Although in one of the experiments SARS-CoV-2 was cultured from feces of confirmed positive patients in the laboratory, still no cases of SARS-CoV-2 infections have been attributed to sewage transmission [52]. The stringency of biological waste treatment also contributes to inactivation of the virus, limiting the amount of infectious virus remaining in these waste streams [53].

Other biological waste materials, such as personal protective equipment (PPE) including masks, gloves, etc., may play roles in the individual-to-individual transmission of SARS-CoV-2. These biowaste materials should be properly segregated according to waste type, and should be subjected to disinfection modalities to minimize the risk of the spread of infection in the environment [54]. For recycling of PPE (gowns, medical gloves, masks and other face and eye shields) waste into value-added products, several advanced processes, such as aminolysis, glycolysis, pyrolysis, hydrogenation, hydrolysis, and gasification are now in practice at the industrial level [55].

Currently, there are only few robust studies that have been reported on reuse of PPE. Thus, the reuse of PPE may harm the healthcare worker via accidental contamination. Therefore, to avoid the possibility of accidental infection, the direct reuse of PPE (i.e., rendering contaminated PPE non-infectious) is not advisable even during acute shortages of PPE [56].

3. Cleaning and disinfection of surfaces for SARS-CoV-2 control

SARS-CoV-2 is transmitted primarily through respiratory droplets and close physical contact. Longer rangee airborne transmission may also occur in hospital areas, due to aerosol-generating medical procedures. Environmental surfaces may act as a source of virus spread in health care settings where certain health care procedures are performed [11, 57]. The virus may be spread via the indirect pathway involving touching of contaminated surfaces followed by touching of susceptible mucous membranes. Alternatively, virus may be re-aerosolized from contaminated surfaces including toilets [58], carpets [59], indoor air [60], fomites [61], etc. Therefore, environmental surfaces such as tables, chairs, light switches, electronic equipment, and toilets, along with medical equipment such as blood pressure cuffs, stethoscopes, etc. must be properly cleaned and disinfected to interrupt the possible transmission of SARS-CoV-2.

SARS-CoV-2 contains a lipid envelope which renders it more susceptible to common disinfectants than non-enveloped viruses, such as rotavirus, poliovirus, etc. [7]. Coronaviruses have been found to be susceptible to the same disinfectants and disinfecting conditions employed to control the risk of several other enveloped viruses. The common disinfection protocols using hydrogen peroxide, sodium hypochlorite, peracetic acid, and UV light that have been employed for the civil and industrial wastewater treatment and inanimate surface hygiene have been found suitable for control of SARS-CoV-2 (**Figure 1**).

SARS-CoV-2 was found to be effectively inactivated by 70% isopropanol, 70% ethanol, 0.1% H_2O_2 and 0.1% sodium laureth sulphate within 60 seconds of exposure on different surfaces, including stainless steel, glass, cardboard, polyvinyl chloride (PVC), polyethylene terephthalate (PET), and cotton fabric [62]. Ethanol and H_2O_2 can conveniently be used for disinfection against SARS-CoV-2 in healthcare settings. Moreover, this study also highlighted the importance of common household detergents (sodium laureth sulphate) and hand soap in rapid inactivation of SARS-CoV-2 [62]. Similarly, in another study, original WHO recommended hand rub formulations I and II [63] and modified formulation I (80% (w/w) ethanol, 0.725% (v/v) glycerol, and 0.125% (v/v) hydrogen peroxide) and formulation II (75% (w/w) 2-propanol, 0.725% (v/v) glycerol, and 0.125% (v/v) hydrogen peroxide) were found effective for reducing SARS-CoV-2 titers to background level within 30 s [64]. Moreover, it is also established that under laboratory conditions >30% (v/v) concentration of 2-propanol and ethanol may also efficiently inactivate SARS-CoV-2 in 30 s [64]. A limitation of alcohol-based disinfectants is the specified

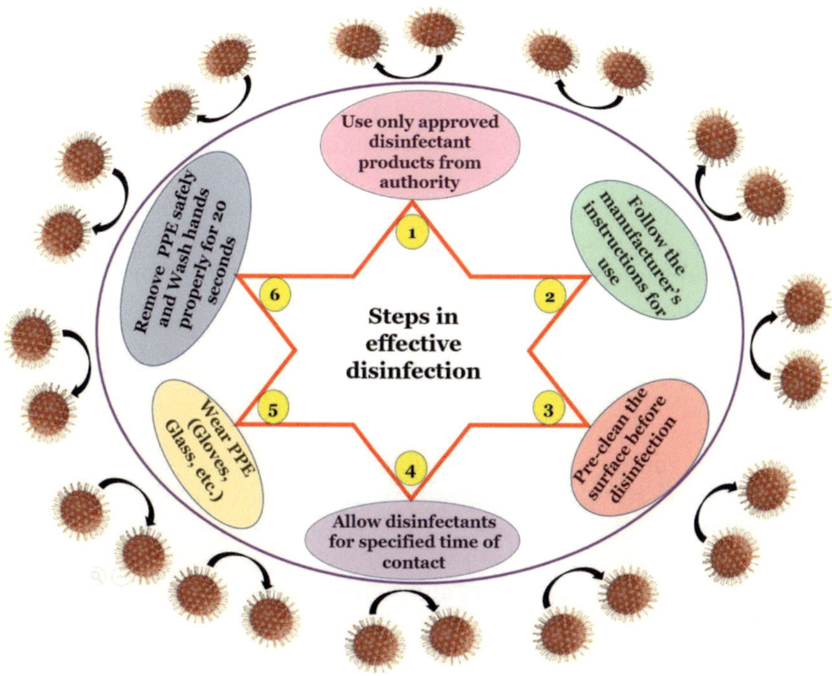

Figure 1.
Steps for application of safe and effective disinfectant against SARS-CoV-2.

inactivation time of exactly 30 s, which must be strictly followed for effective inactivation of virus. In another study, chemical disinfectants including citric acid, quaternary ammonium compounds (QAC), ethanol, and sodium hypochlorite at various concentrations were found effective against SARS-CoV-2 and another associated coronavirus on glass surface. Within a contact time of 0.5 to 10 minutes, these microbicides were able inactivate ≥ 3.0 to ≥ 6.0 $\log_{10}$ [15]. Furthermore, it is a fact that SARS-CoV and MERS-CoV are highly susceptible to disinfectant and detergent treatments, and reports also confirm the susceptibility of SARS-CoV-2 against these chemicals [29]. Therefore, the periodic cleaning and sanitization of HITES should be done to prevent the transmission of SARS-CoV-2. To minimize the adverse impacts of chemical disinfectants on the environment, organizations working in the field of COVID-19 control have recommended the use of microbicides with low environmental impact, such as hydrogen peroxide, phenolic compounds, and hydroalcoholic formulations for COVID-19 control [65].

3.1 Disinfectants for environmental surface cleaning

For surface and environmental disinfection, hypochlorite-based compounds such as powdered calcium hypochlorite and liquid sodium hypochlorite may be used. Upon dissolution in water, these compounds create an aqueous solution of hypochlorous acid (HOCl) as the active antimicrobial ingredient. The HOCl possesses broad spectrum antimicrobial activity against pathogens. A 0.1% (1000 ppm) concentration of hypochlorite is recommended to inactivate the majority of pathogens present in the healthcare areas [66]. However, for blood and bodily fluids, a concentration of 0.5% (5000 ppm) is recommended [67]. Hypochlorite should be freshly prepared before use, because it is rapidly inactivated in the presence of environmental organic material. For better efficacy, surfaces should be thoroughly cleaned with soap or detergent, using mechanical scrubbing or friction, before application of hypochlorite. Hypochlorite should be applied at optimum concentration, because high concentrations of chlorine may lead to metallic corrosion and irritation of skin or mucous membranes. SARS-CoV-2 deposited on HITES can be easily inactivated using chlorine-based disinfectants, detergents, iodine-containing detergents, 70% alcohol, glutaraldehyde, hydrogen peroxide compounds, halogenated compounds, various cationic and anionic surfactants, etc. [68]. SARS-CoV-2 in sewage samples can be effectively inactivated using chlorine dioxide (20 mg/L) [69]. Recently, critical information exploration on predicted and measured virucidal efficacies of several antimicrobial agents against priority viral diseases of WHO, including SARS-CoV-2, have been reviewed by Ijaz et al. [70].

3.2 Spraying of chemical disinfectants and UV irradiation of surfaces in indoor spaces

In indoor areas, routine application of disinfectants by spraying or fogging (i.e., fumigation or misting) is usually not recommended for COVID-19 control because this strategy may not remove all the contaminants outside the spray zones (i.e., not contacted by the spray/fog) [71]. Moreover, fogging using formaldehyde, chlorine-based agents, and quaternary ammonium compounds may also result in risks to the eyes and irritation of the respiratory mucosa or skin [72, 73]. However, some countries have allowed the no-touch methods for applying specific chemical disinfectants, such as vaporized hydrogen peroxide (HPV) in vacated spaces in healthcare settings [74]. In one such experiment, HPV was demonstrated to inactivate >4 $\log_{10}$ of feline calicivirus, transmissible gastroenteritis virus, human adenovirus-1, etc. at lower percentages of active compound (1400 ppm) and lower potential toxicity on living cells [75]. Hydrogen peroxide and 2-phenyl phenol are usually employed for surface disinfection and food sanitation and act as valid alternatives to sodium hypochlorite.

Ultraviolet light irradiation devices have also been modified for use in healthcare settings. Exposure to sunlight or UV light drastically limits coronavirus survival, as is the case for many microorganisms [76]. The efficacy of UV irradiation devices is dependent on several factors, such as irradiation dose, lamp placement, the distance between surface and UV device, wavelength, exposure time, and duration of use, etc. [10] along with fluence of UVC (J/m^2, mJ/cm^2, etc.) which may take into account all other factors [77]. On the basis of review of the UVC inactivation literature, a consensus efficacy of 0.5 to 2 $\log_{10}$ inactivation of SARS-CoV-2 per mJ/cm^2 has been demonstrated. These results indicate that SARS-CoV-2 is quite susceptible to UVC inactivation [24].

In another experiment, more than 3 $\log_{10}$ inactivation of SARS-CoV-2 was detected with a UVC dose of 3.7 mJ/cm^2 on samples contaminated with comparable virus density to that found in COVID-19 patients. However, the complete inactivation of SARS-CoV-2 was observed with 16.9 mJ/cm^2 of UVC [78]. The UV irradiation devices developed for disinfection in health care settings usually are used during terminal surface sanitization i.e., sanitization of rooms after discharge of patient and in rooms unoccupied by the staff and patients. In one of the studies, deep ultraviolet light-emitting diode (DUV-LED) was used for inactivation of SARS-CoV-2 from a COVID-19 patient [79]. Such a study shows the importance of development of DUV-LED based devices to prevent virus contamination of the air and surfaces. However, when using the no-touch disinfection methods, such as fumigation or UV treatment, prior manual cleaning of surfaces is also essential [80]. However, during surface cleaning care should be taken to prevent the re-aerosolization of virus from the surface material, which could represent a potential source of infection. Moreover, for optimal effectiveness, these no-touch approaches should not be considered as replacements for surface cleaning. Rather, after surface disinfection using appropriate virucidal agents, the no-touch approaches can be used to reach surfaces not reached by the surface cleaning methods.

Outdoor application of disinfectants, such as spraying or fumigation on streets and other public places, may not advisable since most of the action of many classes of disinfectant agents are adversely impacted the presence of organic dirt and debris on surfaces. The body surface spraying of individuals with chemical disinfectants in a cabinet, tunnel, or chamber is also not advisable [81]. The research data do not provide evidence of the reduced ability of an infected person, so treated, to spread the virus. Moreover, direct spraying of individuals with a chemical disinfectant, such as a chlorine-releasing agent, may result in irritation in the eye or skin, and may cause nausea, and vomiting, etc. [82, 83].

Healthcare and sanitation personnel involved in disinfection should be provided training in the use of personal protective equipment (PPE) especially in areas where COVID-19 patients are present [84]. Depending upon the disinfectant to be used, healthcare workers involved in the disinfection process should be equipped with a PPE kit including impermeable aprons, face masks, face shields, rubber gloves, and closed shoes [85]. Also, depending upon the disinfectant used, cleaning solutions should be prepared and used in ventilated areas and the mixing of two or more disinfectant solutions should be avoided, because the resultant mixture may be harmful to human health and to surfaces.

3.3 Disinfection in healthcare settings

For environmental cleaning and disinfection of clinical premises, specific international and local authority guidelines should be followed. Surfaces and items with high-touch possibilities, such as door handles, light switches, tables, bed rails, intravenous pumps, etc., should be given proper attention during disinfection. Healthcare workers may act as resource persons for disinfection and cleaning of hospital premises. They should be made aware of cleaning schedules and the risks associated with touching surfaces and equipment during patient care [86]. After a thorough cleaning of environmental surfaces with detergent, 70% alcohol, ≥0.5% hydrogen peroxide, or 0.1% (1000 ppm) to 0.5% (5000 ppm) of chlorine-releasing disinfectants, including sodium hypochlorite, sodium chlorite or chlorine dioxide, can be used for overall disinfection of hospital settings against SARS-CoV-2 [87]. During preparation and application of disinfectants, the use instructions and material safety data sheets supplied by the microbicide manufacturers should be strictly followed to avoid any impacts to humans and to equipment surfaces.

3.4 Disinfection in non-healthcare settings

The risk of fomite (indirect) transmission of SARS-CoV-2 may apply as well to settings outside of hospitals and other healthcare settings. To avoid the risk of any such transmission, it is important to reduce the possibility of contamination in possible high-touch surfaces in offices, homes, schools, gyms, etc. High-touch surfaces in these non-healthcare settings may be thoroughly cleaned with detergent to remove organic dirt and debris before chemical disinfection using sodium hypochlorite (0.1% or 1000 ppm) or alcohol (70–90%) [10].

4. Nanotechnology-based formulations for SARS-CoV-2 control

Although most of the chemical disinfectants are effective against SARS-CoV-2, they are often associated with several drawbacks, such as requirements for higher concentrations for proper virucidal effect, reduced efficacy in the presence of organic substances, and possible risks associated with the environment and public health [88]. The nosocomial transmission through inappropriate PPE may contribute to infection and death of healthcare workers. To prevent nosocomial transmission, PPE can be treated with copper nanoparticles or copper oxides and salts [89]. Nanoparticle-coated non-woven tissues or cloths using metal-grafted graphene oxide (GO) have been found effective against surrogate viruses, including SARS-CoV, MERS-CoV, and Ebola virus [90]. The coating of silver nanoparticles on face masks made up of woven and nonwoven textiles showed efficacy of 99.99% against surrogate viruses for SARS-CoV-2 [91].

Several metallic nanomaterials, such as titanium dioxide, silver, copper, etc. have been proposed as alternatives to chemical-based disinfectants, due to their characteristic antiviral activities, and effectiveness at a much lower concentrations [92]. Nanomaterials act as a virucidal agents via promoting the surface oxidation by toxic ions, leading to inhibition of viral dissemination by inhibiting the binding or penetration of viral particles. The virus penetration to host cells is inhibited by the generation of reactive oxygen species, and photodynamic and photothermal capabilities which destroy the viral membranes [88].

Facial masks coated with silver nanocluster/silica composite showed viricidal effects against SARS-CoV-2 [93]. Similarly, titanium dioxide and silver ion-based nano-formulations can be used for surface disinfection [88]. The cellulose nanofiber-based breathable and disposable filter cartridge may filter particles, including viruses, even those less than 100 nanometers in size [94]. Because of their unique chemical and physical properties, along with a high surface area to volume ratio, some of the nanomaterials such as graphene nanomaterial can be used to adsorb and remove SARS-CoV-2 from surfaces [95]. Graphene-based nanomaterial has been used to make a reusable mask that may trap viruses and inactivate them with the help of an electrical charge [96]. Graphene in association with copper, silver, and titanium nanoparticles, may enhance the antiviral activity and durability of PPE material [90]. Similarly, quaternary ammonium salts, peptides, or polymer-based nanoparticles may promote the oxidation of viral envelopes and inhibit their replication [97]. However, nanomaterials should be used with caution to avoid any possible health hazards. The adverse effects of metallic nanomaterials on the environment and human health can be minimized by utilizing biodegradable nanomaterials, including polymeric lipid-based nanomaterials [98]. However, to the best of available literature, it is difficult to suggest the complete reliance on disinfectant efficacy of nanoparticle-coated PPE, especially against SARS-CoV-2. Hence, traditional chemical-based disinfectants are still primarily in use. However, nano-based formulations represent a promising field of research and will assist in control of current and similar viral outbreaks in the future [99].

5. Conclusion

SARS-CoV-2 may be transmitted through inhalation of virus present in the air farther than six feet away from the source of infection. Apart from airborne transmission, fecal shedding of the virus has been also been reported from some patients. However, the environmental viability of the virus from fecal shedding has been demonstrated at low levels. Moreover, several studies have demonstrated that the environmental survivability of SARS-CoV-2 in wastewater, surface water, sludge, and other biosolid waste material, is very low with temperatures greater than 20°C. Several reports have also demonstrated that the inactivation rate of coronavirus in waste water is higher than other enteric viruses. On inanimate surfaces, SARS-CoV-2 may remain infectious from a few hours to up to a few days. Like most enveloped viruses, SARS-CoV-2 is susceptible to a variety of surface disinfection agents, including ethanol, quaternary ammonium compounds (QAC), sodium hypochlorite, chlorine compounds, etc. Moreover, nanomaterial-based disinfectants have also been investigated for ability to inactivate SARS-CoV-2. Proper public awareness and adequate compliance with recommendations from the public health agencies on appropriate use of personal protective equipment (PPE), adequate application of disinfectants in healthcare settings and public places and the home may reduce the number of infectious SARS-CoV-2 virions on environmental surfaces, which may mitigate the transmission of the virus and the risk of acquiring COVID-19. Moreover, national and international guidelines for infection prevention and control of COVID-19 should be followed strictly and such guidelines should be updated in a timely manner based on new information from the scientific literature.

Acknowledgements

The author is thankful to SVP University of Agriculture and Technology, Meerut, Uttar Pradesh for providing the facility to prepare the manuscript.

Author details

Koushlesh Ranjan
SVP University of Agriculture and Technology, Meerut, Uttar Pradesh, India

*Address all correspondence to: drkoushleshranjan@gmail.com

References

[1] Peeri NC, Shrestha N, Rahman MS, Zaki R, Tan Z, Bibi S, et al. The SARS, MERS and novel coronavirus (COVID-19) epidemics, the newest and biggest global health threats: What lessons have we learned?. International Journal of Epidemiology 2020;**49**(3):717-726. DOI: 10.1093/ije/dyaa033

[2] Geller C, Varbanov M, Duval RE. Human coronaviruses: Insights into environmental resistance and its influence on the development of new antiseptic strategies. Viruses. 2012;**4**(11):3044e3068

[3] Bak A, Mugglestone MA, Ratnaraja NV, Wilson JA, Rivett L, Stoneham SM, et al. SARS-CoV-2 routes of transmission and recommendations for preventing acquisition: Joint British Infection Association (BIA), Healthcare Infection Society (HIS), Infection Prevention Society (IPS) and Royal College of pathologists (RCPath) guidance. The Journal of Hospital Infection. 2021;**114**:79-103. DOI: 10.1016/j.jhin.2021.04.027

[4] Anelich LECM, Lues R, Farber JM, Parreira VR. SARS-CoV-2 and risk to food safety. Frontiers in Nutrition. 2020;**7**:580551

[5] Zhang W, Du RH, Li B, Zheng XS, Yang XL, Hu B, et al. Molecular and serological investigation of 2019-nCoV infected patients: Implications of multiple shedding routes. Emerging Microbes & Infections. 2020;**9**:386-389. DOI: 10.1080/22221751.2020.1729071

[6] Wang S, Tu J, Sheng Y. Clinical characteristics and fecal-oral transmission potential of patients with COVID19. medRxiv. 2020. DOI: 10.1101/2020.05.02.20089094

[7] Rutala WA, Weber DJ. Best practices for disinfection of noncritical environmental surfaces and equipment in health care facilities: A bundle approach. American Journal of Infection Control. 2019;**47**:A96-A105

[8] Sattar SA. Hierarchy of susceptibility of viruses to environmental surface disinfectants: A predictor of activity against new and emerging viral pathogens. Journal of AOAC International. 2007;**90**(6):1655-1658

[9] Chin AWH, Chu JTS, Perera MRA, Hui KPY, Yen H, Chan MCW, et al. Stability of SARS-CoV-2 in different environmental conditions. The Lancet Microbe. 2020;**1**(1):e10. DOI: 10.1016/S2666-5247(20)30003-3

[10] Rutala WA, Weber DJ. Disinfection, Sterilization, and Control of Hospital Waste. Mandell, Douglas, and Bennett's Principles and Practice of Infectious Diseases. 2015;3294-3309.e4. Available from: https://www.ncbi.nlm.nih.gov/pmc/ articles/PMC7099662. DOI: 10.1016/B978-1-4557-4801-3.00301-5

[11] Ong SWX, Tan YK, Chia PY, Lee TH, Ng OT, Wong MSY, et al. Air, surface environmental, and personal protective equipment contamination by severe acute respiratory syndrome coronavirus 2 (SARS-CoV-2) from a symptomatic patient. Journal of the American Medical Association. 2020;**323**(16):1610-1612. DOI: 10.1001/jama.2020.3227

[12] Faridi S, Niazi S, Sadeghi K, Naddafi K, Yavarian J, Shamsipour M, et al. A field indoor air measurement of SARS-CoV-2 in the patient rooms of the largest hospital in Iran. Science of the Total Environment. 2020;**725**:138401. DOI: 10.1016/j.scitotenv.2020.138401

[13] Koh D. Occupational risks for COVID-19 infection. Occupational Medicine. 2020;**70**:3-5. DOI: 10.1093/occmed/kqaa036

[14] Paton S, Spencer A, Garratt I, Thompson KA, Dinesh I,

Aranega-Bou P, et al. Persistence of severe acute respiratory syndrome coronavirus 2 (SARS-CoV-2) virus and viral RNA in relation to surface type and contamination concentration. Applied and Environmental Microbiology. 2021;**87**(14):e0052621. DOI: 10.1128/AEM.00526-21

[15] Ijaz MK, Nims RW, Zhou SS, Whitehead K, Srinivasan V, Kapes T, et al. Microbicidal actives with virucidal efficacy against SARS-CoV-2 and other beta- and alpha-coronaviruses and implications for future emerging coronaviruses and other enveloped viruses. Scientific Reports. 2021;**11**(1):5626. DOI: 10.1038/s41598-021-84842-1

[16] Kasloff SB, Leung A, Strong JE, Funk D, Cutts T. Stability of SARS-CoV-2 on critical personal protective equipment. Scientific Reports. 2021;**11**(1):984. DOI: 10.1038/s41598-020-80098-3

[17] Pastorino B, Touret F, Gilles M, de Lamballerie X, Charrel RN. Prolonged infectivity of SARS-CoV-2 in fomites. Emerging Infectious Diseases. 2020;**26**(9):2256-2257. DOI: 10.3201/eid2609.201788

[18] Matson MJ, Yinda CK, Seifert SN, Bushmaker T, Fischer RJ, van Doremalen N, et al. Effect of environmental conditions on SARS-CoV-2 stability in human nasal mucus and sputum. Emerging Infectious Diseases. 2020;**26**(9):2276-2278. DOI: 10.3201/eid2609.202267

[19] Harbourt DE, Haddow AD, Piper AE, Bloomfield H, Kearney BJ, Fetterer D, et al. Modeling the stability of severe acute respiratory syndrome coronavirus 2 (SARS-CoV-2) on skin, currency, and clothing. PLoS Neglected Tropical Diseases. 2020;**14**(11):e0008831. DOI: 10.1371/journal.pntd.0008831

[20] Liu Y, Li T, Deng Y, Liu S, Zhang D, Li H, et al. Stability of SARS-CoV-2 on environmental surfaces and in human excreta. The Journal of Hospital Infection. 2021;**107**:105-107. DOI: 10.1016/j.jhin.2020.10.021

[21] Riddell S, Goldie S, Hill A, Eagles D, Drew TW. The effect of temperature on persistence of SARS-CoV-2 on common surfaces. Virology Journal. 2020;**17**(1):145. DOI: 10.1186/s12985-020-01418-7

[22] Virtanen J, Aaltonen K, Kivistö I, Sironen T. Survival of SARS-CoV-2 on clothing materials. Advances in Virology. 2021;**2021**:6623409. DOI: 10.1155/2021/6623409

[23] Kampf G, Todt D, Pfaender S, Steinmann E. Persistence of coronaviruses on inanimate surfaces and their inactivation with biocidal agents. The Journal of Hospital Infection. 2020;**104**(3):246-251. DOI: 10.1016/j.jhin.2020.01.022

[24] Nims RW, Plasvic M. Physical inactivation of SARS-CoV-2 and other coronaviruses-a review. In: Nims RW, Ijak MK, editors. Disinfection of Viruses. London, UK: IntechOpen; 2021

[25] van Doremalen N, Bushmaker T, Morris DH, Holbrook MG, Gamble A, Williamson BN, et al. Aerosol and surface stability of SARS-CoV-2 as compared with SARS-CoV-1. The New England Journal of Medicine. 2020;**382**:1564-1567. DOI: 10.1056/NEJMc2004973

[26] Fears AC, Klimstra WB, Duprex P, Hartman A, Weaver SC, Plante KC, et al. Comparative dynamic aerosol efficiencies of three emergent coronaviruses and the unusual persistence of SARS-CoV-2 in aerosol suspensions. medRxiv. 2020. DOI: 10.1101/2020.04.13.20063784

[27] Yepiz-Gomez MS, Gerba CP, Bright KR. Survival of respiratory

viruses on fresh produce. Food and Environmental Virology. 2013;**5**:150-156. DOI: 10.1007/s12560-013-9114-4

[28] Darnell ME, Subbarao K, Feinstone SM, Taylor DR. Inactivation of the coronavirus that induces severe acute respiratory syndrome, SARS-CoV. Journal of Virological Methods. 2004;**121**(1):85-91. DOI: 10.1016/j.jviromet.2004.06.006

[29] WHO. Coronavirus Disease 2019 (COVID-19) situation Report-32 [Internet] 2020. Available from: https://www.who.int/docs/default-source/coronaviruse/situation-reports/20200221-sitrep-32-covid-19.pdf [Accessed: January 28, 2022]

[30] Han J, Zhang X, He S, Jia P. Can the coronavirus disease be transmitted from food? A review of evidence, risks, policies and knowledge gaps. Environmental Chemistry Letters. 2020;**1**:1-12. DOI: 10.1007/s10311-020-01101-x

[31] Liu P, Yang M, Zhao X, Guo Y, Wang L, Zhang J, et al. Cold-chain transportation in the frozen food industry may have caused a recurrence of COVID-19 cases in destination: Successful isolation of SARS-CoV-2 virus from the imported frozen cod package surface. Biosafety and Health. 2020;**2**(4):199-201. DOI: 10.1016/j.bsheal.2020.11.003

[32] Setti L, Passarini F, De Gennaro G, Barbieri P, Perrone MG, Borelli M, et al. Airborne transmission route of COVID-19: Why 2 meters/6 feet of inter-personal distance could not Be enough. International Journal of Environmental Research and Public Health. 2020;**17**(8):2932. DOI: 10.3390/ijerph17082932

[33] Liu Y, Ning Z, Chen Y, Guo M, Liu Y, Gali NK, et al. Aerodynamic analysis of SARS-CoV-2 in two Wuhan hospitals. Nature. 2020;**582**(7813):557-560. DOI: 10.1038/s41586-020-2271-3

[34] Santarpia JL, Rivera DN, Herrera VL, Morwitzer MJ, Creager HM, Santarpia GW, et al. Transmission potential of SARS-CoV-2 in viral shedding observed at the University of Nebraska Medical Center. 2020;**10**(1):12732. DOI: 10.1038/s41598-020-69286-3

[35] Sedlmaier N, Hoppenheidt K, Krist H, Lehmann S, Lang H, Büttner M. Generation of avian influenza virus (AIV) contaminated fecal fine particulate matter (PM(2.5)): Genome and infectivity detection and calculation of immission. Veterinary Microbiology. 2009;**139**(1-2):156-164. DOI: 10.1016/j.vetmic.2009.05.005

[36] Setti L, Passarini F, De Gennaro G, Barbieri P, Perrone MG, Borelli M, et al. SARS-Cov-2RNA found on particulate matter of Bergamo in northern Italy: First evidence. Environmental Research. 2020;**188**:109754. DOI: 10.1016/j.envres.2020.109754

[37] Gundy PM, Gerba C, Pepper IL. Survival of coronaviruses in water and wastewater. Food and Environmental Virology. 2009;**1**(1):10-14

[38] Bivins A, Greaves J, Fischer R, Yinda KC, Ahmed W, Kitajima M, et al. Persistence of SARS-CoV-2 in water and wastewater. Environmental Science & Technology Letters. 2020;**7**(12):937-942. DOI: 10.1021/acs.estlett.0c00730

[39] Rimoldi SG, Stefani F, Gigantiello A, Polesello S, Comandatore F, Mileto D, et al. Presence and infectivity of SARS-CoV-2 virus in wastewaters and rivers. Science of the Total Environment. 2020;**744**:140911. DOI: 10.1016/j.scitotenv.2020.140911

[40] Wigginton KR, Ye Y, Ellenberg RM. Emerging investigators series: The source and fate of pandemic viruses in the urban water cycle. Environmental

Science: Water Research & Technology. 2015;**1**:735-746

[41] Casanova L, Rutala WA, Weber DJ, Sobsey MD. Survival of surrogate coronaviruses in water. Water Research. 2009;**43**(2009):1893-1898

[42] John DE, Rose JB. Review of factors affecting microbial survival in groundwater. Environmental Science & Technology. 2005;**39**(19):7345-7356. DOI: 10.1021/es047995w

[43] Chen C, Hayward K, Khan SJ, Ormeci B, Pillay S, Rose JB, et al. Role of wastewater treatment in COVID-19 control. Water Quality Research Journal. 2021;**56**(2):68-82. DOI: 10.2166/wqrj.2020.025

[44] Wu Y, Guo C, Tang L, Hong Z, Zhou J, Dong X, et al. Prolonged presence of SARS-CoV-2 viral RNA in faecal samples. The Lancet Gastroenterology & Hepatology. 2020;**5**(5):434-435. DOI: 10.1016/S2468-1253(20)30083-2

[45] Medema G, Heijnen L, Elsinga G, Italiaander R, Brouwer A. Presence of SARS_Coronavirus-2 RNA in sewage and correlation with reported COVID-19 prevalence in the early stage of the epidemic in the Netherlands. Environmental Science & Technology Letters. 2020;**7**(7):511-516. DOI: 10.1021/acs.estlett.0c00357

[46] Peccia J, Zulli A, Brackney DE, Grubaugh ND, Kaplan EH, Casanovas-Massana A, et al. SARS-CoV-2 RNA concentrations in primary municipal sewage sludge as a leading indicator of COVID-19 outbreak dynamics. 2020:1-12. DOI: 10.1101/2020.05.19.20105999

[47] Nabi G. Detecting viral outbreaks in future using enhanced environmental surveillance. Environmental Research. 2020;**188**:109731. DOI: 10.1016/j.envres.2020.109731

[48] Wang XW, Li JS, Guo TK, Zhen B, Kong QX, Yi B, et al. Concentration and detection of SARS coronavirus in sewage from Xiao Tang Shan hospital and the 309th hospital. Journal of Virological Methods. 2005;**128**(1-2):156-161. DOI: 10.1016/j.jviromet.2005.03.022

[49] Ding Z, Qian H, Xu B, Huang Y, Miao T, Yen HL, et al. Toilets dominate environmental detection of severe acute respiratory syndrome coronavirus 2 in a hospital. Science of The Total Environmen. 2021;**753**:141710. DOI: 10.1016/j.scitotenv.2020.141710

[50] Haji Ali B, Shahin MS, Masoumi Sangani MM, Faghihinezhad M, Baghdadi M. Wastewater aerosols produced during flushing toilets, WWTPs, and irrigation with reclaimed municipal wastewater as indirect exposure to SARS-CoV-2. Journal of Environmental Chemical Engineering. 2021;**9**(5):106201. DOI: 10.1016/j.jece.2021.106201

[51] Duan SM, Zhao XS, Wen RF, Huang JJ, Pi GH, Zhang SX, et al. SARS research team. Stability of SARS coronavirus in human specimens and environment and its sensitivity to heating and UV irradiation. Biomedical and Environmental Sciences. 2003;**16**(3):246-255

[52] Zhang Y, Chen C, Zhu S, Shu C, Wang D, Song J, et al. Isolation of 2019-nCoV from a stool specimen of a laboratory-confirmed case of the coronavirus disease 2019 (COVID-19). China CDC Weekly. 2020;**2**(8):123-124

[53] Wolff MH, Sattar SA, Adegbunrin O, Tetro J. Environmental survival and microbicide inactivation of coronaviruses. In: Schmidt A, Wolff MH, Weber O, editors. Coronaviruses with Special Emphasis on First Insights Concerning SARS. Basel/Switzerland: Birkhauser Verlag; 2005

[54] Iyer M, Tiwari S, Renu K, Pasha MY, Pandit S, Singh B, et al. Environmental survival of SARS-CoV-2 - a solid waste perspective. Environmental Research. 2021;**197**:111015. DOI: 10.1016/j.envres.2021.111015

[55] Siwal SS, Chaudhary G, Saini AK, Kaur H, Saini V, Mokhta SK, et al. Key ingredients and recycling strategy of personal protective equipment (PPE): Towards sustainable solution for the COVID-19 like pandemics. Journal of Environmental Chemical Engineering. 2021;**9**(5):106284. DOI: 10.1016/j.jece.2021.106284

[56] Gov.uk. [WITHDRAWN] Considerations for acute personal protective equipment (PPE) shortages [Internet] 2022. Available from: https://www.gov.uk/government/publications/wuhan-novel-coronavirus-infection-prevention-and-control/managing-shortages-in-personal-protective-equipment-ppe [Accessed: January 28, 2022]

[57] Ye G, Lin H, Chen L, Wang S, Zeng Z, Wang W, et al. Environmental contamination of the SARS-CoV-2 in healthcare premises. The Journal of Infection. 2020;**81**(2):e1-e5. DOI: 10.1101/2020.03.11.20034546

[58] Dancer SJ, Li Y, Hart A, Tang JW, Jones DL. What is the risk of acquiring SARS-CoV-2 from the use of public toilets? The Science of the Total Environment. 2021;**792**:148341. DOI: 10.1016/j.scitotenv.2021.148341

[59] Haines SR, Adams RI, Boor BE, Bruton TA, Downey J, Ferro AR, et al. Ten questions concerning the implications of carpet on indoor chemistry and microbiology. Building and Environment. 2020;**170**:106589. DOI: 10.1016/j.buildenv.2019.106589

[60] Ijaz MK, Zargar B, Wright ICE, Rubino JR, Sattar SA. Generic aspects of the airborne spread of human pathogens indoors and emerging air decontamination technologies. American Journal of Infection Control. 2016;**44**:S109-S120

[61] Stephens B, Azimi P, Thoenunes MS, Heidarinejad M, Allen JG, Gilbert JA. Microbial exchange via fomites and implications for human health. Current Pollution Reports. 2019;**5**:198-213

[62] Gerlach M, Wolff S, Ludwig S, et al. Rapid SARS-CoV-2 inactivation by commonly available chemicals on inanimate surfaces. The Journal of Hospital Infection. 2020;**106**(3):633-634. DOI: 10.1016/j.jhin.2020.09.001

[63] WHO. WHO guidelines on hand hygiene in health care: first global patient safety challenge clean care is safer care [Internet] 2009. Available from: https://apps.who.int/iris/bitstream/handle/10665/44102/9789241597906_eng.pdf [Accessed: January 28, 2022]

[64] Kratzel A, Todt D, V'kovski P, Steiner S, Gultom M, Thao TTN, et al. Inactivation of severe acute respiratory syndrome coronavirus 2 by WHO-recommended hand rub formulations and alcohols. Emerging Infectious Diseases. 2020;**26**(7):1592-1595. DOI: 10.3201/eid2607.200915

[65] WHO. Laboratory biosafety guidance related to the novel Coronavirus (2019-nCoV) [Internet] 2020. Available from: https://www.who.int/docs/default-source/coronaviruse/laboratory-biosafety-novel-coronavirus-version-1-1.pdf. [Accessed: January 28, 2022]

[66] Sangkham S. Face mask and medical waste disposal during the novel COVID-19 pandemic in Asia. Case Studies in Chemical and Environmental Engineering. 2020;**2**:100052. DOI: 10.1016/j.cscee.2020.100052

[67] CDC. Best Practices for Environmental Cleaning in Healthcare

Facilities: in Resource-Limited Settings, version 2. [Internet] 2019. Available from: https://www.cdc.gov/hai/pdfs/resource-limited/environmental-cleaning-RLS-H.pdf. [Accessed: January 28, 2022]

[68] Lin Q, Lim JYC, Xue K, Yew PYM, Owh C, Chee PL, et al. Sanitizing agents for virus inactivation and disinfection. View (Beijing). 2020;**24**:e16. DOI: 10.1002/viw2.16

[69] Totaro M, Badalucco F, Costa AL, Tuvo B, Casini B, Privitera G, et al. Effectiveness of disinfection with chlorine dioxide on respiratory transmitted, enteric, and Bloodborne viruses: A narrative synthesis. Pathogens. 2021;**10**(8):1017. DOI: 10.3390/pathogens10081017

[70] Ijaz MK, Nims RW, Cutts TA, McKinney J, Gerba CP. Predicted and measured virucidal efficacies of microbicides for emerging and reemerging viruses associated with WHO priority diseases. In: Disinfection of Viruses. London, UK: InTech Open; 2022

[71] Roth K, Michels W. Inter-hospital trials to determine minimal cleaning performance according to the guideline by DGKH, DGSV and AKI. Zentr Steril. 2005;**13**(2):106-116

[72] Mehtar S, Bulabula ANH, Nyandemoh H, Jambawai S. Deliberate exposure of humans to chlorine-the aftermath of Ebola in West Africa. Antimicrobial Resistance and Infection Control. 2016;**5**:45. DOI: 10.1186/s13756-016-0144-1

[73] Schyllert C, Rönmark E, Andersson M, Hedlund U, Lundbäck B, Hedman L, et al. Occupational exposure to chemicals drives the increased risk of asthma and rhinitis observed for exposure to vapours, gas, dust and fumes: A cross-sectional population-based study. Occupational and Environmental Medicine. 2016;**73**:663-669. DOI: 10.1136/oemed-2016-103595

[74] Weber DJ, Rutala WA, Anderson DJ, Chen LF, Sickbert-Bennett EE, Boyce JM. Effectiveness of ultraviolet devices and hydrogen peroxide systems for terminal room decontamination: Focus on clinical trials. American Journal of Infection Control. 2016;**44** (Suppl. 5):e77-e84. DOI: 10.1016/j.ajic.2015.11.015

[75] Goyal SM, Chander Y, Yezli S, Otter JA. Evaluating the virucidal efficacy of hydrogen peroxide vapour. The Journal of Hospital Infection. 2014;**2014**(86):255-259

[76] Patel M, Chaubey AK, Pittman CU Jr, Mlsna T, Mohan D. Coronavirus (SARS-CoV-2) in the environment: Occurrence, persistence, analysis in aquatic systems and possible management. Science of The Total Environment. 2021;**765**:142698. DOI: 10.1016/j.scitotenv.2020.142698

[77] Malayeri AH, Mohseni M, Cairns B, Bolton JR. Fluence (UV dose) required to achieve incremental log inactivation of bacteria, protozoa, viruses and algae. IUVA News. 2016;**18**:4-6

[78] Biasin M, Bianco A, Pareschi G, Cavalleri A, Cavatorta C, Fenizia C, et al. UV-C irradiation is highly effective in inactivating SARS-CoV-2 replication. Scientific Reports. 2021;**11**(1):6260. DOI: 10.1038/s41598-021-85425-w

[79] Inagaki H, Saito A, Sugiyama H, Okabayashi T, Fujimoto S. Rapid inactivation of SARS-CoV-2 with deep-UV LED irradiation. Emerging Microbes & Infections. 2020;**9**(1):1744-1747. DOI: 10.1080/22221751.2020.1796529

[80] Rutala WA, Weber DJ. Disinfectants used for environmental disinfection and new room decontamination technology. American Journal of Infection Control.

2013;**41**:S36-S41. DOI: 10.1016/j.ajic.2012.11.006

[81] WHO. Cleaning and disinfection of environmental surfaces in the context of COVID-19. 2020. Available from: https://www.who.int/publications/i/item/cleaning-and-disinfection-of-environmental-surfaces-inthe-context-of-covid-19 [Accessed: January 25, 2022]

[82] Zock JP, Plana E, Jarvis D, Antó JM, Kromhou H, Kennedy SM, et al. The use of household cleaning sprays and adult asthma: An international longitudinal study. American Journal of Respiratory and Critical Care Medicine. 2007;**176**:735-741. DOI: 10.1164/rccm.200612-1793OC

[83] Benzoni T, Hatcher JD. Bleach Toxicity, in: StatPearls. Treasure Island (FL): StatPearls Publishing; 2020. Available from: https://www.ncbi.nlm.nih.gov/books/NBK441921

[84] Medina-Ramon M. Asthma, chronic bronchitis, and exposure to irritant agents in occupational domestic cleaning: A nested case-control study. Occupational and Environmental Medicine. 2005;**62**:598-606

[85] Yates T, Allen J, Leandre Joseph M, Lantagn D. WASH Interventions in Disease Outbreak Response. Oxfam; Feinstein International Center; United Kingdom: UKAID; 2017. DOI: 10.21201/2017.8753

[86] Gon G, Dancer S, Dreibelbis R, Graham WJ, Kilpatrick C. Reducing hand recontamination of healthcare workers during COVID-19. Infection Control and Hospital Epidemiology. 2020;**41**(7):870-871. DOI: 10.1017/ice.2020

[87] Ying Liu X, Zhang Y, Tu HX, Leck A. Cleaning and disinfection in health care settings during the COVID-19 outbreak. Community Eye Health. 2020;**33**(109):36-37

[88] Talebian S, Wallace GG, Schroeder A, Stellacci F, Conde J. Nanotechnology-based disinfectants and sensors for SARS-CoV-2. Nature Nanotechnology. 2020;**15**(8):618-621. DOI: 10.1038/s41565-020-0751-0

[89] Sportelli MC, Izzi M, Kukushkina EA, Hossain SI, Picca RA, Ditaranto N, et al. Can nanotechnology and materials science help the fight against SARS-CoV-2? Nanomaterials. 2020;**10**(4):802. DOI: 10.3390/nano10040802

[90] Bhattacharjee S, Joshi R, Chughtai AA, Macintyre CR. Graphene modified multifunctional personal protective clothing. Advanced Materials Interfaces. 2019;**6**(21):1900622. DOI: 10.1002/admi.201900622

[91] Abulikemu M, Tabrizi BEA, Ghobadloo SM, Mofarah HM, Jabbour GE. Silver nanoparticle-decorated personal protective equipment for inhibiting human coronavirus infectivity. ACS Applied Nano Materials. 2022;**5**:309-317. DOI: 10.1021/acsanm.1c03033

[92] Bratovcic A. Available recycling solutions for increased personal protective equipment in the environment due to the COVID-19 pandemic. Aswan University Journal of Environmental Studies. 2021;**2**(1):1-10. DOI: 10.21608/aujes.2021.57293.1009

[93] Weiss C, Carriere M, Fusco L, Capua I, Regla-Nava JA, Pasquali M, et al. Toward nanotechnology-enabled approaches against the COVID-19 pandemic. ACS Nano. 2020;**14**(6):6383-6406. DOI: 10.1021/acsnano.0c03697

[94] El-Atab N, Mishra RB, Hussain MM. Toward nanotechnology-enabled face masks against SARS-CoV-2 and pandemic respiratory diseases. Nanotechnology. 2021;**33**(6):1-22. DOI: 10.1088/1361-6528/ac3578

[95] Palmieri V, Papi M. Can graphene take part in the fight against COVID-19? Nano Today. 2020;**33**:100883. DOI: 10.1016/j.nantod.2020.100883

[96] De Maio F, Palmieri V, Babini G, Augello A, Palucci I, Perini G, et al. Graphene nanoplatelet and graphene oxide functionalization of face mask materials inhibits infectivity of trapped SARS-CoV-2. iScience. 2021;**24**(7): 102788. DOI: 10.1016/j.isci.2021.102788

[97] Campos EVR, Pereira AES, de Oliveira JL, Carvalho LB, Guilger-Casagrande M, de Lima R, et al. How can nanotechnology help to combat COVID-19? Opportunities and urgent need. Journal of Nano biotechnology. 2020;**18**(1):125. DOI: 10.1186/s12951 020-00685-4

[98] Su S, Kang PM. Systemic review of biodegradable nanomaterials in Nanomedicine. Nanomaterials. 2020;**10**(4):656. DOI: 10.3390/ nano10040656

[99] Ikner LA, Gerba CP. Antiviral coatings as continuously active disinfectants. In: Nims RW, Ijak MK, editors. Disinfection of Viruses. London, UK: IntechOpen; 2021